More praise for *The End of Illness*

"David Agus, one of the nation's most innovative cancer doctors, shatters the myths about health and wellness and provides us with a handbook for living a long, healthy life."

—Steve Case, chairman of Revolution and
The Case Foundation; cofounder America Online

"In this seminal book, Dr. David Agus presents a brilliant new model of health based on the body as a complex system with an emphasis on prevention. *The End of Illness* may reframe everything you thought you knew about health. It is both provocative and inspiring. Highly recommended."

—Dean Ornish, MD, founder and president of the
Preventive Medicine Research Institute; clinical professor of medicine
at the University of California, San Francisco

"David Agus is one of the great medical thinkers of our age. *The End of Illness* reframes the entire discussion of sickness and health. Instead of thinking about disease, Agus thinks about the system that is the human body, and what we need to do to guide it toward health. Before you take your next vitamin, read this book."

—Danny Hillis, PhD, cofounder, Applied Minds and Thinking Machines

"Dr. David Agus has been disrupting medicine as we know it for his entire career. Now he brings his ideas out of the lab and exam room and into the lives of everyone—showing us how to live long, healthy, disease-free lives. Reading this book is the best thing you can do for yourself and your loved ones. A monumental work that will change your life."

—Marc Benioff, chairman and CEO, salesforce.com

*f*P

THE END OF ILLNESS

David B. Agus, MD
with Kristin Loberg

Free Press
New York   London   Toronto   Sydney   New Delhi

613
A

NOTE TO READERS

Free Press
A Division of Simon & Schuster, Inc.
1230 Avenue of the Americas
New York, NY 10020

First Free Press hardcover edition January 2012

FREE PRESS and colophon are trademarks of Simon & Schuster, Inc.

For information about special discounts for bulk purchases, please contact Simon & Schuster Special Sales at 1-866-506-1949 or business@simonandschuster.com

The Simon & Schuster Speakers Bureau can bring authors to your live event. For more information or to book an event contact the Simon & Schuster Speakers Bureau at 1-866-248-3049 or visit our website at www.simonspeakers.com.

Designed by Carla Jayne Jones

Manufactured in the United States of America

10 9 8 7 6

Library of Congress Cataloging-in-Publication Data

Agus, David, 1965–
   The end of illness / by David Agus.
      p. cm.
   1. Health.   2. Diseases—Causes and theories of causation.   I. Title.
RA776.5.A38   2011
613—dc23   2011034347

ISBN 978-1-4516-1017-8
ISBN 978-1-4516-1020-8 (ebook)

"It doesn't take a hero to order men into battle. It takes a hero to be one of those men who goes into battle."

—Norman Schwarzkopf, United States Army general and commander of U.S. Central Command, retired; prostate cancer survivor and advocate

To my patients throughout the years.
It's an honor and privilege to be a part of your care.
This book is as much yours as it is mine.
Thank you for being my heroes.

The part can never be well unless the whole is well.

—Plato

Contents

Contents

THE END OF
ILLNESS

Introduction

Notes from the Edge

How a Cancer Doctor Met His Greatest Challenge to End All Illness

> If you wish for peace, understand war.
>
> —*B. H. Liddell Hart in* Strategy *(1967)*

Over the last two decades, I have developed a unique way of looking at the relationship of the human body to health and disease. It has enabled me to challenge people's most guarded, rational convictions on health. Perhaps this is the result of what I've been doing for these past twenty years or so—fighting on the front lines as a cancer doctor and researcher. I feel as if I've been dangling out on the edge of a cliff with fellow physicians searching for better treatments to this ravaging disease that claims more lives today than it should. Cancer treatment is the place where we take the most risks in medicine because, frankly, there's little hope for survival in many cases, and the cure is as evasive today as it ever was.

1

I'm infuriated by the statistics, disappointed in the progress that the medical profession has made, and exasperated by the backward thinking that science continues to espouse, which no doubt cripples our hunt for the magic bullet.

Now, with this book, I'm taking a moment to step away from that ledge and share what I've learned, which has everything to do with all things health-related. It's like that old saying of having to go to war to understand peace. The war on cancer might be ugly and destructive on many levels, but on a positive note there are many lessons learned in the experience of this war that can then be used to prevent future wars and maximize peace. After all, the goal should be to avoid ever having to go to war, rather than to win a war. And in the health realm, this is especially true.

Some of you may not be battling cancer, but my guess is you'd like to steer clear of it. You'd also like to know how to achieve the seemingly intangible goal of "health" in your life—to maximize your body's peaceful well-being. Much in the way my job enables me to break certain "rules" to test out new theories about cancer, this book breaks "rules" with the same intention: to potentially save lives. I have a hunch that just as I've triggered a mix of curiosity, disbelief, wonder, and sometimes anger when I present my ideas to audiences, I'll be doing the same here, but, again, it's all for good reason: to prolong your life and help you to make every year a better one. Put simply, what you're going to find is unlike what's in any other book you've ever read in the health category—or any category, for that matter. It's part manifesto, but it's also part life plan.

Take a moment to imagine what it would be like to live robustly to a ripe old age of one hundred or more. Then, as if your master switch clicked off, your body just goes kaput. You die peacefully in your sleep after your last dance that evening. You don't die of any particular illness, and you haven't gradually been wasting away under the spell of some awful, enfeebling disease that began years or decades earlier. Most of us can't picture ourselves avoiding the ailments that tend to end others' lives prematurely and sometimes suddenly. Yet I want you to believe that you can live a long, fulfilling, disease-free life—because it is possible. The end of illness is closer than you might think. It is my wish for you. But to achieve this superhuman feat, you have to understand health from a new perspective and embrace a few tenets of well-being that probably go against everything you've ever learned.

I'm going to presume that you're a pretty reasonable, levelheaded individual. You follow the news and keep abreast of the latest health and medical studies making headlines. You try to remember to take your daily multivitamin and find time to exercise. Perhaps you worry about pollution, pesticides, and the quality of the water streaming through your faucets. You also know somewhere deep down that you should bank more restful sleep at night, eat more fresh fruits and vegetables, and trim more saturated fat from your diet. But what if I told you that you weren't necessarily right on these universal principles? What if everything you thought about health was *wrong*?

What *is* health? It seems like a simple question for which there is a simple answer. Is it a number, such as weight or cholesterol level? Or is it a lifestyle—being an active person and eating "healthily"? I wish it were that straightforward. In an era where the explosion of medical information has far outstripped our ability to process it, we need a new way to make personal health choices. If you come to me for help in treating advanced cancer detected late in the game, your game is likely to be over soon. I don't say this unaffectionately or to sound insensitive; I say it because it's the truth. I'm a realist, and the facts of cancer and many other life-threatening diseases are unnerving. In an age when we can communicate in seconds with people around the world using slick devices we tote in our pockets, it's a shame that the technology and innovation in medical research and treatment are so archaic, outdated, and, dare I say, in some cases barbaric.

My intent in putting this book together is threefold: (1) to propose a new model of health that will dramatically change your view of the human body; (2) to show you how to apply that model to your own life through tactical strategies and practical prescriptions; and (3) to reveal eye-opening medical technologies that are currently available or in development that can help you to achieve the quality of life and longevity that you deserve. With the information disclosed in this book, you'll commence a journey down a completely different path from the one you're on now, and it will change your life for the better.

Forewarning: Some of the topics I will cover and the advice I will suggest may make you uncomfortable at first. You will learn facts and become immersed in concepts that may go against everything that you've been taught or conditioned to believe is "right" or "healthy." My thoughts on what makes a human well or, conversely, *unwell* may not follow established ways of thinking. In that regard, this book is a manifesto in the truest sense of the word—a bold declaration that paints an untraditional picture of the body and its vast mechanisms that drive it either interminably toward or away from health.

The central premise of the book is that, for decades, we—all of us, whether you're part of the health-care community or not—have been thinking about health and our bodies in an incorrect manner. We've tried to whittle our understanding of the body and its afflictions down to a single point—be it a mutation, a germ, a deficiency, or a number such as blood pressure or blood glucose. Rather than honoring the body as the exceedingly complex system that it is, we keep looking for the individual gene that has gone awry or for the one "secret" that can improve our health. This kind of shortsightedness has led us far astray from an essential perspective that we'll be exploring in this book, and which will not only change how we take care of ourselves, but also how we spur the next generation of treatments and, in some instances, cures. It has also caused us doctors to betray the very oath we took—"do no harm"—when we recited Hippocrates upon getting our degrees. Because the truth is that some doctors inflict a lot of harm today. The entire notion of "do no harm" has been corrupted; we've moved to an extreme place in medicine that's rarely data-driven and is horrendously overrun by false or unproven claims. And that's scary.

A Systems View Is Born

In 2004, while walking from Cedars-Sinai Hospital to my clinic in L.A., my eyes scanned the gift shop's window where the cover of the latest *Fortune* magazine shouted out to me, "Why We're Losing the War on Cancer." The story had been penned by cancer survivor Clifton Leaf, whose life had been saved by a clinical trial when he was a teenager in the 1970s. It left a deep impression on me, for any cancer doctor who comes across such a blunt headline and well-thought-out essay is bound to feel disheartened and failing at his most essential job. After Clifton was diagnosed with Hodgkin's disease, his parents drove him to upstate New York from the city so he could receive what was an experimental therapy at the time: a brutal protocol involving MOPP, the first combination of chemotherapy drugs to treat the condition successfully. He was subjected to a ping-pong regime of chemotherapy alternating with radiotherapy, which led to the removal of his thyroid after accidental irradiation. But his treatment rendered a cure, and he would go on to become a crusader for the cancer community. Now a keynote or featured speaker at the major scientific conferences around the world, Clifton adds a refreshing, passionate voice to the conversation as both an award-winning journalist and fierce patient advocate whose goal is to set the priorities straight.

Clifton made remarkable points in the article, the most significant of which explained how we—as a society, but more specifically, within the medical community—have come to look at biology. For the last fifty years, we have focused on trying to understand the individual features of cancer in order to treat it rather than putting our efforts directly into *controlling* cancer. We have forgotten that curing cancer starts with preventing cancer, and that detecting cancer in its earliest stages is critical if people are going to have a chance to preempt or control the disease before it enters that deadly stage of malignancy. When we reduce science down to the goal of finding the tiniest improvements in treatment rather than genuine break-throughs, we lose sight of the bigger picture and find ourselves lost.

Is this why we've barely budged in our "war" against cancer in the last five decades? Does this explain the widening gap between advancing cancer treatments and other therapies for all kinds of ill-nesses? Gnawing questions like these began to bother me. I am, after all, an oncologist who cannot treat advanced cancer well. Med-ical science has made extraordinary progress over the past century, but in my field, the progress stalled out decades ago.

Our outlooks on life may evolve slowly over time, but they can shift in an instant when a new fact or finding is brought to our at-tention. My perspective on health began to take a serious turn when I read Clifton's article, and then it crystallized one night in the company of a Nobel laureate in physics who pushed me to think differently. In July 2009, I attended a dinner party in Aspen, Colo-rado, where I had the good fortune of meeting Murray Gell-Mann, the scientist who had postulated the existence of quarks nearly fifty years previously. Quarks, particles more elementary than electrons, are the basic building blocks of all matter in the universe. We owe much of our understanding of how the universe organizes itself at the subatomic level to Murray's work. He received the 1969 Nobel Prize in physics even though his concepts weren't confirmed until 1977.

Murray couldn't have been a more engaging and charming fellow for his seventy-nine years, with an infectious smile to boot. I had an immediate intellectual crush on his zest for life and brilliancy, and I was eager to hear about Murray's theoretical endeavors in the physical sciences. Like thoughts, you cannot see a quark using the most advanced technologies, and when Murray was initially coming up with his ideas, he had to rely on discrete sets of data and infer from those that quarks must exist. My aha moment came when he talked about the complex systems he confronted in physics and how he would go about trying to build models to understand those systems. Why hadn't doctors approached medicine like this? Why didn't we try to do something similar with all the sets of data we collect and come up with a model to understand illness and, conversely, health? Just as Murray could describe his quark model, I sought to define an analogous model for the medical field, and I came up empty. The word *oncologist* literally means "one who studies masses, or tumors." Murray defined certain (albeit subatomic) masses in terms of physics, while I was attempting to understand biological masses associated with abnormality and chaos. I began to wonder how I could apply Murray's way of thinking to my own world.

Since that night, I've had the privilege of exchanging ideas with Murray on numerous occasions (and I'm fortunate that he has joined my research team part-time as a Presidential Professor of Physics and Medicine at the University of Southern California so that we can work more closely together). Despite the generations between us, we get along like old friends. As much as we admire one another's fields of work, we are also intrigued by how each of our professions has groomed us to think differently. When Murray said to me point-blank, "Look at cancer as a *system*," I really began to rethink everything—about cancer and our approach to treating it; about illness and our approach in medicine in general; and ultimately, about health. I couldn't help but ask myself: Is our way of looking at cancer keeping us from curing it? Moreover, does this faulty perspective preclude us from treating *anything* in medicine successfully?

As I'll explain in this book, I firmly believe in trying to identify cancer early. Catching cancer early is currently the only way we can effectively fight it. If we follow certain health rules, we are able, in fact, to prevent most cancers. But this notion doesn't just pertain to cancer. We can actually stave off many illnesses and diseases through targeted preventive measures, and that's what this book is about.

Let me be clear: this is not a "cancer book." Rather than thinking of cancer only as a major disease and formidable enemy, we should think about cancer as a metaphor for the basket of the world's Illnesses with a capital I. Cancer is the most advanced of all the diseases we can put in this basket. It's not an outlier. As Siddhartha Mukherjee writes, it's the "emperor of all maladies"—the ultimate nemesis that hangs in the balance for one in three women and one in two men during their lifetime. We've got a serious problem on our hands if all the intelligence and money currently going toward cancer are doing next to nothing in this so-called war. It's time to change not only how we think about cancer, but also how we think in broader terms of health and wellness. We need a radically different way of thinking that can lead to breakthroughs in all areas of medicine. This new way of thinking entails a new way of caring for our bodies and defining what health means on each of our own terms, for health is not just the absence of disease.

A Career of Questions

I've been interested in human biology for as long as I can remember. As a kid I was interested in the sciences early on, and I embraced the laboratory at a young age. I've had many remarkable mentors through the years, including my physician father, who always set the bar high for me, encouraging me to stay curious. When the time came to decide what type of doctor I'd become, following a stint at the National Institutes of Health and then Johns Hopkins Hospital, I was told that being an oncologist was "career suicide." The advice was to enter cardiology or pulmonary medicine, where you could "make a difference." No one went from a residency at Hopkins to a place such as the Memorial Sloan-Kettering Cancer Center in New York City to study cancer, which at the time was an insipid branch of medicine bereft of hope and innovation. As if it were yesterday, I can vividly recall the clinical leaders at Hopkins asking me why I wanted to go into a field that gave poison to patients with little or no benefit. I saw it differently and followed my heart to become a lymphoma doctor before getting involved with prostate cancer research, clinical care, and drug and technology development. I didn't believe that oncology was a dead end. Much to the contrary, it was one of the few areas in medicine where doctors and patients abandoned tradition and took risks to arrive at better treatments because there were so few options. I wanted to apply solutions discovered in the lab to disease right away and participate in the future of cancer medicine.

In the late 1990s, I founded Oncology.com, the largest Internet cancer resource and community at the time. My adventures were just beginning. When Andy Grove, the former CEO and chairman of Intel and one of my dearest mentors, nudged me to move West, he knew I was seeking to do something different. I still remember May 13, 1996, the day Andy bravely appeared on the cover of *Fortune* magazine to talk about his diagnosis and treatment for prostate cancer, which had been a hushed-about illness for far too long. Inspired by my many talks with him and the entrepreneurism on the West Coast, I moved my young family to California, where I began to forge the kinds of connections that would help me make good on my ambitions as a young boy learning the ropes in a laboratory. I cofounded Applied Proteomics and Navigenics, two health-care technology and wellness companies (whose technologies I'll explain later in this book); and I took on leadership roles at prominent institutions including Cedars-Sinai Medical Center, UCLA, and USC. I had a feeling that the future of medicine would rely on a marriage between technology and biology, and that I'd have to engage in a wide variety of projects across a range of industries that would link back to my ultimate mission: to change patients' outcomes and have an impact on the role of illness in our lives. It is this mission that has brought me to realize that we've veered off track in our thinking about health—and how to reclaim it.

In This Book

Originally, the title for this book was *What Is Health?* This title was intended to be a play on the acclaimed physicist Erwin Schrödinger's *What Is Life?*, a book published in 1944 directed at the lay reader to explain the body's innate drivers of life. But I quickly abandoned using the word *health* in the title after a friend said bluntly in an e-mail, "To me, *health* sounds like something I'm supposed to eat but tastes really bad." His response to my potential title idea demonstrates the very problem I'm attacking. Our present concept and understanding of health have evolved to so much of a "he said, she said" nature that we have forgotten what it's all about. I hope with this book to set the record straight and refocus energy and resources toward a new definition of health.

One of the most important messages of the book is that there is no "right" answer in health decisions; rather, there are several right answers. You have to make the right decisions for you—based on your personal code of values and health circumstances, and in consultation with your own physician. My job in these pages is to empower you with understanding so you can make the best decisions for yourself. In doing so, I'll be addressing questions that you likely never thought to ask. For example:

- How can a simple peek at your body's proteins tell you more about the state of your health this instant than a readout of your genetic code?

- What do statins such as Lipitor and Crestor have in common with the swine flu and Alzheimer's disease?
- Which two lifesaving products do officials from the Centers for Disease Control and Prevention carry with them everywhere they go, which you can buy for under $10 at Wal-Mart?
- Do some of our most treasured promoters of health such as vitamins, supplements, and even drinks made by juicing fruits and vegetables disrupt the body's preferred state of being?
- How can a drug that never touches a cancerous cell eradicate an entire colony of cancerous cells?
- If you're looking to preserve your health, happiness, and longevity, what's the single most important thing you can do today that costs absolutely nothing?

In other words, what have we been missing when it comes to decoding the mystery of disease? And, in turn, what will define your path to vibrant, long-lasting health?

I'm going to answer those questions. To do this requires an exercise in thought and perspective: you have to embrace the body as a uniquely complex creature and redefine health on your own terms using what I call "metrics" to measure the state of your health regularly. I will propose the various ways in which you can establish your metrics and personalize your medical care. A glass of red wine a day, for instance, may enhance the health of your best friend but put you at a higher risk for certain cancers. Many of the "prescriptions" detailed in this book are surprisingly practical, such as wearing comfortable shoes and eating lunch at the same time every day. Along the way, I'm also going to push you to rethink many sacred cows, such as the idea that low vitamin D should be remedied with supplements and that a one- or two-hour workout in the morning makes up for sitting most of the day. I'll be dismantling myths and misinformation in the hope that I will inspire you to take actionable steps today that will help you lead a healthier life starting right now.

Unlike what you might find in typical diet books, which take you day by day, meal by meal, calorie by calorie, my recommendations won't be terribly exacting. I'm not interested in telling you how to live your life or what you should be eating for dinner. I'm also not here to diagnose you. Instead, I want to empower you to take control over your body and the future of your health. The suggestions offered here are more like lifestyle algorithms—mental devices for thinking through our myriad lifestyle choices. Those choices must be tempered by our values and individual codes of ethics and behavior. Because there is no single answer to the question of what is health, these guidelines will produce as many different "healthy styles" as there are people living them.

My objective is to help you make the most of your health, whether or not you're currently battling an illness. I'd like to encourage you to take a hard look at your understanding of health and open up your mind to a change in perspective. It can significantly improve your life.

That we need simple reminders of what it means to live a healthy life despite the volume of advice transmitted daily in the media is a telling sign of our confusion. I can only hope that as you read this book you gain not only the knowledge you need to take advantage of modern science and medicine, but also the wisdom to discern the good from the questionable to make the best decisions for yourself. I also hope that your future will be determined by the power of choice, and, when necessary, that it will guide you down pathways of healing. Only you can end illness.

PART I

The Science and Art of
Defining Your Health

I f I had to sum up this entire book in a single phrase, it would be this: get to know yourself. I don't mean that in a cosmic or purely psychological way. I'm a big believer in what's called personalized medicine, which refers to customizing your health care to your specific needs based on your physiology, genetics, value system, and unique conditions. We are finally entering an exciting time in medicine where we have the technology to custom-tailor treatment and preventive protocols just as we'd custom-tailor a suit or designer gown to one's individual body. But it all begins with you. You have to know yourself in a manner that you've probably never done before.

Right now, most of us live by sweeping, general guidelines that are one-size-fits-all. If you want to lose weight, for example, you pick a diet that's marketed to everyone and which likely recommends that you eat more fibrous vegetables and cut back on processed sugar. If you want to reduce your risk for cancer, you'll be told to avoid tobacco smoke, to exercise regularly, and to take early detection seriously. But imagine being able to have a more explicit oracle into your future health, as well as a more exacting set of rules to follow today. Think about what it would be like, for instance, to know precisely how to tweak your diet to effortlessly lose twenty pounds for good, or to have a detailed list of things to avoid and things to embrace that make you feel fantastic and be in tip-top shape, or to know what the perfect amount of medicine X is for you to combat affliction Y successfully with no side effects. That's the promise that personalized medicine has to offer.

But, once again, you won't be able to enjoy the benefits of personalized medicine until you get up close and personal with yourself. Nothing about health is one-size-fits-all, so until you know how to perform your own "fitting," you won't be able to live the long and happy life that's awaiting you.

The checklist below used to be buried deep in the book somewhere—long after I'd done a lot of explaining and storytelling—but I've since plucked it out and placed it here. I want to give you a first step in the right direction before I spend a couple hundred pages fleshing out all of my recommendations in detail. This questionnaire was originally designed to help you prepare for a checkup with your doctor, giving you clues to discuss during your visit. However, while piecing this book together, I realized that the same questionnaire should be filled out before even reading the book, which will help you to know yourself better before embarking on this adventure. I also know that you want to be told what to do as soon as possible, and even though you'll find lots of "health rules" to consider throughout this book, many of which will be called out at the ends of chapters, at least the following questions will equip you with concepts to think about as you read further and incorporate my advice into your life. This questionnaire is also downloadable online at www.TheEnd ofIllness.com/questionnaire, where you'll find a version that you can respond to directly on the page to print for your records and/or take to your doctor.

Personal Health Inventory Questionnaire

- *Overall feeling:* How do you feel? It's arguably the most important question to ask of yourself. You might feel great today, but how about yesterday? When do you have your low moments? Is there a pattern? Is it hard for you to get out of bed in the morning?
- *Energy levels:* How would you rank your energy level on a scale of 1 to 10? How has it changed in the last year?
- *Schedule:* How regular is your schedule of when you eat, exercise, and sleep? Is every day the same or different?
- *Breathing:* Anything abnormal to report? Do you hear or feel rattles when you breathe? Does it hurt to breathe deeply? Do you cough when you take a deep breath? Answer these questions when you are at rest and after exercise.
- *Exercise tolerance:* How much can you comfortably tolerate? How does this amount of physical activity compare with how you felt and how hard you moved your body last year? Does anything hurt or feel funny when you move or exercise?
- *Walking:* Are you walking the same way you always have? Do you lean to one side and never did before? Do you hunch over more? Is it hard to walk fully upright?
- *Sensations:* Anything unusual or out of the ordinary to report in any part of your body? For example, how is your sense of smell? Is it as strong as ever? Weak?
- *Skin:* When you scan your skin for any strange marks, growths, or bumps while naked in front of the mirror, do you find anything? Has anything changed since the last time you examined your skin? Do your socks leave indentation marks on your ankles/legs? (If so, this could

indicate that your heart isn't working properly and fluid is getting stagnant in areas, increasing your risk for a blood clot.)

- *Hair:* Has your hair changed at all in terms of thickness, texture, growth/loss, and so on? Have you lost hair around your ankles? This could be a sign of a circulatory problem, especially noticeable in men. Conversely, do you have hair growing in odd places, such as your arms and face? This could signal hormonal changes, especially in women.

- *Nails:* These dead tissues can actually tell you a lot. Have they changed in appearance or color lately? Discolored nails can signal certain conditions, from a simple infection to diabetes. If your nails have a yellowish hue to them, it's time for a diabetes check. Nails can also indicate iron levels. Look for a whitish crescent C at the base of your nails, which indicates good iron levels.

- *Fingers:* Do your joints ache after using them? If you're a woman, is your ring finger longer than your index finger? If so, you may be twice as likely to suffer from osteoarthritis. That's according to a 2008 study in the journal *Arthritis & Rheumatism*, which discovered this odd connection and hypothesized that longer ring fingers are linked to higher levels of testosterone exposure in the womb. Higher prenatal levels of testosterone lower the concentration of estrogen, which is critical to bone development. If you're a man whose index finger is longer than your ring finger, your risk of prostate cancer drops by a third.

- *Joints:* Do they hurt? More in the morning when you get up, or after a long day? What makes the aching joints better?

- *Appetite:* Is it the same as it used to be? Stronger? Weaker? Do you have serious cravings? If so, for what?
- *Breasts:* If you're a woman, do you see or feel any lumps, bumps, or dimples when you perform a breast exam?
- *Digestion:* Any feelings of discomfort to report? Do you have to use any over-the-counter medications for your digestion/stomach on a regular basis (e.g., Tums, Pepto-Bismol, Tagamet, Zantac, Prevacid, laxatives, and the like)? If you have symptoms, are they better or worse after eating a meal? Do you experience an intolerance, sensitivity, or allergy to certain foods?
- *Headaches:* Do you experience headaches regularly? Migraines? Do you know the triggers for such headaches? Do you find yourself taking over-the-counter painkillers consistently (e.g., Advil, Aleve, Tylenol, Excedrin, aspirin, and the like)?
- *Allergies:* Do you have any? Have your allergies changed over the years? How so?
- *Sleep:* Do you sleep well? Do you resort to sleep aids on occasion? Do you wake up feeling rested most of the time? How consistent are your bedtimes and wake times? Does your bed partner say that you snore? (Sleep apnea, which is often characterized by snoring, is incredibly common today and is a known risk factor for a heart attack. Luckily, sleep apnea can be treated pretty successfully.)
- *Pain:* Is there any area where you feel discomfort or pain?
- *Passing colds and flus:* Do you get sick a lot? How many fevers have you had this past year? When you get sick, does it seem to take you longer than your friends or family members to get better? Did you get a flu shot this year?

- *Mood*: How stable is your mood? Do you have feelings of depression?
- *Hormonal cycle*: If you're a woman, is your cycle regular? Are you in perimenopause or menopause?
- *Previous diagnoses*: What have you previously been diagnosed with? Is there anything that you deal with chronically?
- *Stress level*: On a scale of 1 to 10, how bad is it? Is it chronic or just once in a while? Does the stress affect your lifestyle? If your stress is work-related, do you love or hate your job? (Turns out that if you love your job despite the stress, you're much better off than if you hate your job and it causes you stress!)
- *Weight*: Are you happy with it? Have you tried to change it? What happened when you did? Do you have a paunch that you cannot get rid of?
- *Medications (prescription and nonprescription)*: What do you take, for what conditions, and for how long have you been taking them? This includes all vitamins, supplements, additives, and occasional medications (such as a few Tylenol or Advil for a headache).
- *Health-care prevention*: Are you up-to-date with things like routine exams/wellness checkups, vaccines, screenings (e.g., Pap smear, colonoscopy, etc.), and blood tests? Do you know what foods you're supposed to be eating given your underlying disease risk factors?
- *Overall satisfaction*: If you had to rank how you felt about yourself in general, on a scale of 1 to 10, what would your number be? What kind of report card would you give yourself? What do you want to change in your life?

Unlike other self-tests you find in books and magazines, this one doesn't have a scorecard at the end. Your answers are your own. Once you've incorporated some of my forthcoming suggestions, come back to this questionnaire to check in with yourself whenever you want. See how you change from month to month and year to year. Continue to ask yourself, am I as healthy as I want to be?

Part I is all about defining your health, and I'll begin by taking you on a tour of how we've lost our compass with respect to understanding the human body. I'll reveal a new perspective that gives us a more accurate compass, and then I'll help you to use that compass in your journey to optimize your health with the technology we have today. At the end of Part I, I'll share one of the most powerful medical technologies currently in development that will soon allow each of us to personalize our medicine in a truly sophisticated manner. Knowing about this technology now will give you hope for the future, as well as add context to the information in the rest of the book.

1

What Is Health?

A New Definition That Changes Everything

Everyone has a vague idea of what it means to live a healthy life. Eating a balanced diet: good. Smoking: bad. Breaking a sweat regularly: good. Binge drinking: bad. Getting a restful night's sleep: bonus. Being happy: double bonus. Some of us may choose to disregard these basic tenets on occasion, but for the most part, we know the difference between the habits that help us stay youthful and strong, and those that can detract from our well-being.

We try our best to stay out of harm's way, but what happens when we get sick or develop a chronic medical condition or, heaven forbid, are diagnosed with a serious illness? After experiencing the frustration of *Why me?* many of us begin to ask ourselves other, more probing inquiries about where we might have gone wrong. Was it something in the water? A lifelong love of hamburgers and fries? An overdemanding boss and, as a result, an overwhelming stress level?

Too much alcohol? Too little exercise? Secondhand smoke? Exposure to industrial chemicals? A habit of living dangerously, whatever that might mean? Bad luck?

Or perhaps, some of us think, this outcome was fated because it was just *in my DNA all along.*

If I could collect a nickel for every time someone in the world thought that genetics was wholly to blame for this illness or that defect, I'd be the wealthiest man on earth. It's human nature to point fingers at someone or something else for our flaws and shortcomings, and to avoid any personal culpability. Because DNA tends to be a relatively abstract construct, much like black holes or quarks, which we cannot touch, see, or feel, it might as well be a "something else" to which we can assign guilt. After all, DNA is "given" to us by our parents and we have no choice. In this regard, DNA is practically accidental; just as accidents happen, so does DNA, without our having much say in the matter.

What most people don't think about, though, is that DNA says more about our risk than our fate. It governs probabilities, not necessarily destinies. As my friend and colleague Danny Hillis (whom we'll meet later when I cover emerging technologies) likes to describe it, DNA is simply a list of parts or ingredients rather than a complete manual that explains how those parts work together to generate results. To hold your DNA responsible for your health is missing the forest for the trees. It's not the pièce de résistance. I say this knowing full well that DNA does hold certain keys to your health; if it didn't, then I wouldn't have cofounded a company that performs genetic testing so you can take preventive measures based on your genomic risk profile. But right from the get-go I want to entice you to start thinking from a broader perspective that goes far beyond your genes. I want you to view your body—from the outer stretches of your skin to the inner sanctum of your cellular makeup—as a whole system. It's a uniquely organized and highly functioning system that leaves so much to the imagination because we're only just beginning to solve its riddles.

So therefore, as we probe the mystery of the human body more deeply, we discover that this system, and its complex riddles, don't necessarily hinge on DNA alone.

The Inescapable Statistics

To understand how we've arrived at a place where we focus so much on DNA, and why it's critical to respect the body as an elaborate system beyond genetics, it helps to explore the evolution of our thinking processes against the backdrop of the challenges we've faced—and continue to face—in our quest for health and longevity.

Most of our transformative breakthroughs in medicine have occurred only recently, in the last sixty or so years. Following the discovery of penicillin in 1928, which changed the whole landscape of fighting infections based on the knowledge that they were caused by bacteria, we got good at extending our lives by several years and, in many cases, decades. This was made possible through a constellation of contributing circumstances, including a decline in cigarette smoking, changes in our diets for the better, improvements in diagnostics and medical care, and of course advancements in targeted therapies and drugs such as cholesterol-lowering statins.

Heart disease has been the leading cause of death in the United States since 1921, and stroke has been the third-leading cause since 1938; together, these vascular diseases account for approximately 40 percent of all deaths. Since 1950, however, age-adjusted death rates from cardiovascular disease have declined 60 to 70 percent, representing one of the most important public health achievements of the twentieth century.

Death Rates for Leading Causes of Death: All Ages

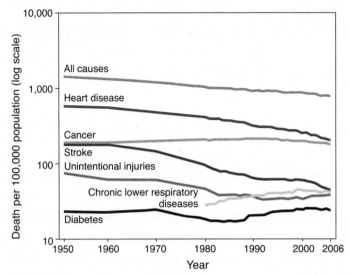

Age-adjusted data.
Source: CDC/NCHS, *Health, United States, 2009*, Figure 18. Data from the National Vital Statistics System.

Put another way:

Change in US Death Rates* by Cause, 1950 to 2007
Rate per 100,000

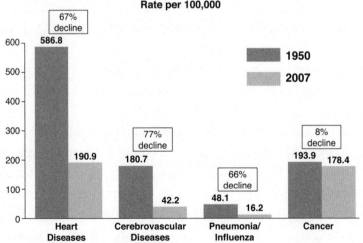

*Age-adjusted to 2000 US standard population.
Source: 1950 Mortality Data - CDC/NCHS, NVSS, Mortality Revised.
2007 Mortality Data – National Center for Health Statistics, Centers for Disease Control and Prevention, 2010.
http://www.cdc.gov.

But here's the sobering truth sitting on the sidelines of these triumphs like a lumbering white elephant: the death rate from cancer from 1950 to 2007 (the most current data available from the Centers for Disease Control and Prevention) didn't change much. We are making enormous progress against other chronic diseases, but little against cancer. Indeed, there are little wins here and there with unique types of cancer. Take, for instance, chronic myelogenous leukemia, a rare type of leukemia that had previously been a death sentence except for a small number of patients who benefited from bone-marrow transplantation. With the FDA approval of Gleevec (brand name for imatinib mesylate) in May 2001—the same month it made the cover of *Time* magazine as the "magic bullet" to cure cancer—we now have a way to successfully treat most patients and achieve remarkable recovery rates. The drug targets the particular chromosomal rearrangement that is present in this disease (part of chromosome 9 is fused to part of chromosome 22). In clinical trials, the response rate to Gleevec was over 90 percent. People went from their deathbeds to functional life after taking this small molecule with few side effects. But with the more common deadly cancers, including those that ravage the lung, colon, breast, prostate, brain, and so on, we've had an embarrassingly small impact on death rates.

Whenever I throw the chart on the previous page, "Change in the US Death Rates by Cause," on a slide up in front of an audience, I hear a few gasps of disbelief. How can this be? What did we do wrong in our research? Is there is mistake, or perhaps a typo, in this data? I showed this graphic during my 2009 TEDMED talk as part of a larger discussion that included thirty-seven other slides and have received hundreds of e-mails since referring to just this one slide. Many of the inquiries are aggressive in tone—accusing me of being a pessimist and somehow manipulating the data. I wish I could present better news from my camp.

This graph demonstrates the profound effect that therapeutics such as statins have had in heart disease and stroke. Antibiotics and antivirals, including vaccines, have put a major dent in cases of pneumonia and infections. Even when we consider cancer rates across the globe, we can find some statistics that defy all the stereotypes. In some of the sub-Saharan countries, where we tend to think about diseases such as AIDS and other infections common in underdeveloped nations, more people die of cancer than of HIV, tuberculosis, and malaria *combined*. In 2010, chronic disease overtook infectious disease as the leading killer worldwide. So this problem isn't just a major cause of concern in America. It affects the global community at large.

The lack of change in the death rate from cancer is truly alarming. The more astonishing observation that I want you to note here, though, is that antibiotics and antivirals do not target the human being—they target the external, invading organism. Statins, on the other hand, target the human system in ways that we are starting to learn more about. Contrary to popular belief, the statins work not just by lowering cholesterol through a single pathway or point of interaction in the body; they have a profound effect on the entire system, lowering inflammation, thereby changing the body's entire environment. Vaccines also target the system, but do so in a clever way—activating the immune system artificially by making it seem as though a foreign organism has invaded the body.

I stated plainly in the introduction that this isn't a cancer book, but I need to draw from my experience as an oncologist to get you to understand a few core concepts. We can actually trace our relationship to health to the study of cancer. When we consider the legacy of disease in our history and how we've come to understand today a mysterious malady such as cancer, we can begin to see how and why we may have veered off track. We can identify the thinking processes and misconceptions that we've blindly embraced and that have thwarted our efforts to advance medicine and, in turn, our individual goals of optimal health. On a positive note, we can begin to see how we can shift direction and embrace a new frontier in the pursuit of health customized to each person, you and me. We can eventually reach a point where we can make meaningful advances in the "war" against all illnesses.

A Cancerous Perspective

Cancer, as I explained earlier, is a great metaphor for anything related to sickness. It's every person's archenemy, the bearer of all things "bad" when it comes to health, happiness, and of course longevity. All of us fear learning that our body has turned against us—that cancer has struck and the future is uncertain. This uncertainty can be most unpleasant. Suddenly we cannot answer questions such as where, how, why, and when—as in *when will I be cancer-free?* Or, *when will I die?*

The most insidious part of cancer is the very nature of this beast: it's self-generated in the sense that it's our own

What is cancer? If you have a mass or an abnormal blood test, you'll likely be referred to a specialist who will stick a needle in you and extract a sample to be examined by a pathologist. Your pathologist (whom you will probably never meet) will look for a certain pattern, because diagnosis today is by pattern recognition. Does it look *normal*? Or does it look *abnormal*?

To make an analogy, consider a plastic water bottle as emblematic of a cell. It's as if your pathologist is looking at a normal plastic bottle and declaring that it's a normal cell. And then looking at a deformed, crushed plastic bottle and declaring that it's a cancer cell. That is the state of the art today in diagnosing cancer. There's no molecular test. There's no sequencing of genes. There is no fancy examination of the chromosomes. This is how we do it.

cells gone awry. There's no outside invader. No foreign organism or contagion with a mind of its own and a cellular makeup unlike ours. Cancer is like a sleeping giant lying dormant in all of us. Sometimes, he briefly awakens, inciting a collection of odd cells called a tumor,

27

but, in most cases, before long he's tamed and lulled back to sleep by the body's arsenal of artful mechanisms. But occasionally, often when we least expect it, this giant manages to get past our trusty gatekeepers. Something in our defense mechanisms breaks down, throwing off the checks and balances that came so automatically and reliably before, and this causes cellular dysfunction that leads to the growth of cancerous tumors. Cancer presents certain challenges not present in other illnesses, especially those that can easily be blamed on outsiders. Still, the question remains, why can't we make headway in understanding and combatting cancer, however small and slow?

In 2009, I stood before thousands of colleagues at a meeting of the American Association for Cancer Research in Denver and bluntly said, "We've made a mistake." We've all made a mistake, myself included, by focusing down, by reducing the study of disease down to finite points. I proposed that we take a big step back, take a twenty-thousand-foot view of disease. I then made another statement that ruffled a few more feathers in the room: "We don't necessarily need to understand cancer to control it." The hisses that I heard leaking from the audience were somewhat disheartening. People evidently got upset, but it was critical to call out where we'd strayed as doctors—and as members of society—because this could help get us back on track. I was as guilty as anyone else in this straying. I didn't leave this particular audience hanging, though. I knew I had to provide some explanation to justify my statements and offer at least some hope for the future. I then shared how we had grown accustomed to a certain mode of thinking in the sciences that owes its origins to discoveries made a long time ago.

We've had a hard time moving past the germ theory of disease, which dominated, and in many ways defined, medicine in the twentieth century. According to this theory, if you can figure out what species of germ you are infected with, then your problem is solved because that tells you how you should treat the disease. This became the general paradigm of medicine. Doctors would perform a laboratory test to determine what the infectious agent was, then apply a treatment that was specific for that agent or class of agents. The treatment only cared about the invading organism, such as the bacterium that causes tuberculosis or the parasite that leads to malaria; it didn't care to define or understand the host (the human being) or even where the infection was happening in the host. That is why we use the same drug in every patient with a particular infectious disease.

Which is precisely what doctors try to do: identify the disease—diagnose—and treat the diagnosis according to the best-known method. This strategy also allows science to participate because it can objectively test whether a particular treatment is effective when dealing with a given diagnosis. Does quinine help the symptoms of malaria? Is penicillin the best way to treat anthrax? Once science proves what's best, that's what the doctors do. Diagnose. Treat. Diagnose. Treat. We, as patients hoping that science makes headway in improving our health, must question these methods and ask ourselves if there's another, better way—especially for diseases of our system, such as heart disease and cancer, rather than diseases with invading organisms such as the infectious ones.

This scientific approach to medicine is relatively new. Historically, doctors had theories that resembled the traditional Hindu system of ayurvedic medicine, with its emphasis on balances between various forces in the body. Or in the West, a medieval doctor might have tried to make you less "choleric" or more "phlegmatic." Like Eastern philosophies, the idea was to try to restore the order of the various forces that were controlling the body. But this approach to medicine and honoring the body as a whole was all but abandoned in the early twentieth century, especially in the West, where we became distracted by our triumph over infectious agents. It's all the more interesting to note that, at the time that the germ theory of disease was really exploding and antibiotics were being discovered, renowned geneticist J. B. S. Haldane articulated the following at Cambridge on February 4, 1923:

The recent history of medicine is as follows. Until about 1870 medicine was largely founded on physiology, or, as the Scotch called it "Institutes of Medicine." Disease was looked at from the point of view of the patient, as injuries still are. Pasteur's discovery of the nature of infectious disease transformed the whole outlook, and made it possible to abolish one group of diseases. But it also diverted scientific medicine from its former path, and it is probable that, were bacteria unknown, though many more people would die of sepsis and typhoid, we should be better able to cope with kidney disease and cancer. Certain diseases such as cancer are probably not due to specific organisms, whilst others such as phthisis [a term for tuberculosis no longer used] are due to forms, which are fairly harmless to the average person, but attack others for unknown reasons. We are not likely to deal with them effectually on Pasteur's lines, we must divert our view from the micro-organism to the patient. Where the doctor cannot deal with the former, he can often keep the patient alive long enough to be able to do so himself. And here he has to rely largely on a knowledge of physiology. I do not say that a physiologist will discover how to prevent cancer. Pasteur started life as a crystallographer. But whoever does so is likely at least to make use of physiological data on a large scale. The abolition of disease will make death a physiological event like sleep. A generation that has lived together will die together.

Haldane summed up his thoughts and simultaneously made an extraordinary prediction when he stated, in reference to the germ theory, "This is a disaster for medicine because we're going to get focused on these germs, and we're going to forget about the system." He was completely right nearly ninety years ago! Indeed, as a society, and as people desperately looking for culprits to blame for our health woes, we began to make assumptions. We started to assume that our ills originated from the outside world, which was the absolute wrong assumption to make when it came to afflictions that had nothing to do with germs and had everything to do with our *inside* world.

The Genetics of Infectious Thinking

The germ theory spelled disaster for treating illnesses such as cancer because scientists and laypeople alike started thinking of them almost as if they were infectious diseases. It became a habit of thought that then established how people were treated, and which continues to this day. So when patients visit their doctor, they are diagnosed and placed in a category—e.g., diabetes versus celiac disease—and then they receive the treatment that is shown to work on that category of diagnosis—e.g., insulin control versus avoidance of gluten. In the case of cancer, doctors treat it like an invader and try to cut it out or poison it. The exact treatment protocol depends on which body part is involved, such as the breast or prostate.

But cancer isn't nearly as straightforward as infectious diseases. Diagnosing, categorizing, and treating make a lot of sense for infectious diseases because infections are species—they speciate and divide out, and as such need to be treated like the invaders that they are. In the case of an infectious disease, be it caused by a virus or a bacterium, if we target the Achilles' heel of the intruder, we win. We don't need to know anything about the host; we just need to know who the intruder is and how to kill it. The problem also becomes one of scale: with infectious disease, we only need to consider one scale—the virus or bacterium. But with other human diseases, we need to consider multiple scales, such as the diseased cell, the organ it involves, other nearby organs, the whole body, and so on. It's no longer a one-on-one battle where one side just needs the right gun. It's an inscrutable morass of battles, some of it resembling a small civil war and some of it echoing a large war crossing borders.

Now, to understand the complexity with which a disease such as cancer spreads and how it bears no resemblance to infectious disease, let's look at how the National Cancer Institute describes cancer on its website*:

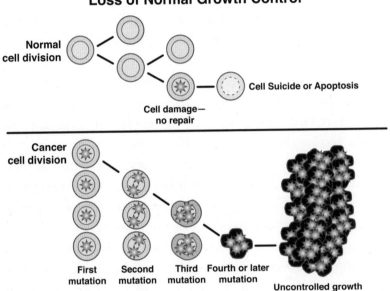

Loss of Normal Growth Control

The illustration does a decent job of conveying how cells divide and that at the heart of the matter is a cancerous cell's increased cell growth rate or inability to commit suicide. But this depiction tells only part of the story, leaving out a crucial component.

For much of history, we didn't know what caused cancer or why tumors developed, but we had a vague hunch that cancer was related to a systemic problem—a profound bodily dysfunction that could not necessarily be solved by surgery or poison.

---

*http://www.cancer.gov/cancertopics/understandingcancer/cancer/page4

Though some people like to opine that cancer is a modern disease and that the sins of our industrial world—directing blame at pollution, fast and processed food, and environmental toxins—are what fuel an alleged surge in cancer rates, I don't subscribe to this line of thinking. I agree that cancer is often seen as symbolic of our modern culture of abundance, excess, and overproduction, but cancer is as old as the human race and has been documented since ancient history. Seven Egyptian papyri written between 3000 and 1500 BC describe syndromes consistent with our description of cancer. One in particular, the Edwin Smith Papyrus, named after the man who procured or pilfered this fifteen-foot-long papyrus from an antiques seller in Luxor, Egypt, in 1862, describes eight cases of tumors or ulcers of the breast. Written likely in the seventeenth century BC, the document states that no treatment is known for this condition and recommends cauterization, using a hot instrument to burn it out. Today's surgery and radiation therapy are similar to the described cauterization; all that's changed is we now have sharper knives and thankfully anesthesia. The ancient Egyptians developed different protocols for benign and malignant tumors. This included surgical removal of "surface tumors." For malignant tumors, they referred to a list of compounds to treat these more problematic manifestations of the disease. Barley, castor oil, and animal parts such as the pig's ear were all suggested. The oldest physical evidence of cancer can be found in the skull of a woman from the Bronze Age, between 1900 and 1600 BC. The tumor is similar to what we would presently describe as a head-and-neck cancer. We also have the mummified remains of a Peruvian Inca that's 2,400 years old that shows the undeniable signs of melanoma.

Flash forward a few thousand years, during which cancer undoubtedly continued to ravage human bodies of old and young. Among the most insightful and observant of early physicians in more recent ancient history was the Roman physiologist, surgeon, and writer Galen, who proposed theories on illness and disease at a time when numerous scientific disciplines such as anatomy, pathology, and pharmacology were still in their infancy. Practicing medicine in the second century, Galen contributed a substantial amount to the Hippocratic understanding of pathology. Hippocrates, you might recall from your high school biology days, is considered the father of medicine and established many cogent theories on health during the classical Athens period, around 400 BC. His physiological and philosophical observations became the foundation upon which modern medicine is based, for he is credited with being the first person to believe that diseases were caused naturally and not as a result of superstition and gods. Moreover, his writings first described the difference between malignant and benign tumors. Detailing cancer by body part, Hippocrates named the disease *karkinos*, which is Greek for "crab," to describe tumors that progress to ulceration.

It's hard to see how cancer can look like a crab, but the crab image was an appropriate one for Hippocrates. The tumor that Hippocrates sought to describe had a bunch of inflamed blood vessels around it, which made him think of a crab buried in the sand with its legs splayed in a circle. That Hippocrates came to describe cancer as looking like a crab clearly indicates that he wasn't looking at the kinds of cancers that we cannot see with the visible eye. He was observing mostly large tumors close to or on the body's surface such as those of the breast, skin, neck, and tongue.

Hippocrates's thoughts on health and disease allowed future protégés such as Galen to expand and experiment on his concepts, some of which perceptively hinted at the definition of cancer. Galen described cancer as being intractably and inexorably part of the whole body. According to Galen, a glut of widespread "black bile" rooted cancer firmly and could not be easily extracted or done away with. This black bile invaded the entire body, with tumors reflecting the extensiveness and stubbornness of this permeating malignant state. Attempts to cut out these tumors could be met with resistance, as the black bile would not only fill in that hole but also foster another tumor. Galen may have lacked the sophisticated vocabulary and instruments such as gene sequencers and microscopes that we have today, but he was spot-on in his descriptions of cancer's systemic qualities and its ability to pervade, proliferate, and regenerate.

Many of Galen's theories endured until the Renaissance period, and medical students continued to study Galen's writings until well into the nineteenth century. Then, when nineteenth-century pathologists focused their microscopes on these invasive cellular masses, they discovered the cruel joke that defines cancer: it's our own cells in excess, not "black bile" in overabundance. But these cells might as well be black bile because they act like rebellious blobs that break boundaries and sack other tissues. What they have in common with other cancerous cells is not only an abnormal shape but also rampant cellular proliferation—runaway cell growth under no control. Siddhartha Mukherjee describes this process beautifully in his book *The Emperor of All Maladies*, which paints a rich historical picture of cancer in the biography of humankind.

On the molecular level, cancer happens after changes to cellular genes. Normal cells are equipped with powerful genetic signals that instruct when and how cells can divide to create more cells. Some genes activate cellular propagation, acting like little accelerators of growth. Others behave like molecular brakes, halting growth. This explains why, for example, when a skin wound heals, the cells involved in the mending know when to stop producing new cells so you're not left with clumps of extra skin. But in a cancer cell, this brilliant balance between active growth and inactivity is disrupted. The green and red lights that normally control the traffic of growth are misfiring and generating too many green lights. The cell is then left without its regulator and doesn't know how to stop growing.

But this molecular view of cancer isn't all that helpful in coming up with treatments because to me, cancer looks like the following:

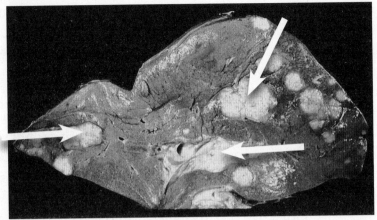

a) Human liver with cancer that originated in the colon.

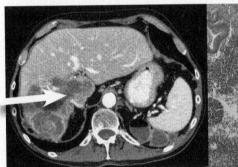

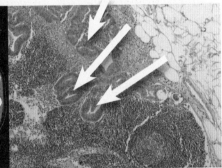

b) A computerized axial tomography (CAT) scan showing cancer in the liver.

c) A microscopic image of cancer in the lymph node.

Here we have (a) a liver with colon cancer, what I'd technically call "colon cancer metastatic to the liver"; it has traveled—metastasized—from the colon to the liver, evidenced by the white masses; (b) a CAT scan of another liver with colon cancer invading it ("colon cancer metastatic to the liver"; note the five circular, dark masses on the left side of the image); and (c) a microscopic image of colon cancer in a lymph node ("colon cancer metastatic to lymph node"). To clarify, if you have "colon cancer" that travels to the lungs, it doesn't become "lung cancer." It's still colon cancer—and looks like colon cancer.

Cancer is an interaction of a cell that is no longer under growth control within the environment. What's even more important to grasp is that cancer isn't just about uncontrolled cell division and the proliferation of a cellular clan; it's about another critical characteristic that embodies cancer: its ability to evolve over time. Although people like to envision cancer as a static mad cellular copying machine, it's much more clever and dynamic than that. Every time a new generation of cancer cells is born, those cells harbor new mutations—mutations that go beyond those already present in the genes that are supposed to regulate growth. Making matters worse, when cancer is exposed to chemotherapy, drug-resistant mutants can escape. In other words, just as resistant strains of bacteria can result from antibiotic use, anticancer drugs can produce resistant cancer cells.

But again, let's move past the molecular view of cancer for a moment. As you can see from looking at cancer, evolution selects for cancer's *appearance*, not its genetics. Yes, cancers all have different genes, but they all look alike. There may be fifty different molecular ways to arrive at a particular body "cancer," such as breast, colon, lung, brain, or prostate, but they all appear and act the same way in the end. If I showed a pathologist ten breast cancers from ten different patients, the molecular underpinnings of each would be totally different, yet they would all look like breast cancer under the microscope. By the same token, there'd be a striking similarity between the look of breast cancer cells and cancerous cells from any other organ in the body because cancerous cells have a lot in common in appearance and behavior. This is a key point in comprehending cancer. Scientists have long focused on the molecular defects to cancer—not what it actually looks like. The National Cancer Institute's diagram of cancer on page 32 gets only part of the story. Cancer isn't a disease of the genes. Rather, it's a disease where cells evolve to look and behave a certain way, using gene alterations to get there. So while we may find a way to block one molecular pathway in our attempts to treat the disease, that doesn't mean cancer can't find its way down another path, which it usually does in an efficient fashion, unfortunately.

Consider someone you know who has cancer. That person used to be somebody who didn't have cancer, and he or she still has the same DNA in the cells of the body. The difference between having cancer and not having cancer doesn't solely reside in the genome. Most of that person's cells are not turning into cancer. Cancer is a dynamic process that's happening, and it's happening far from the confines of a static piece of DNA. Now, a specific mutation from a genome may help explain why it started. For instance, one of the exceptional genetic-test successes has been in breast cancer, which has found BRCA1 and 2, specific genes that are associated with a high risk for breast cancer. Mutations in this gene are more common in Ashkenazi Jews, but it's important to understand that a mutation in BRCA1 and BRCA2 doesn't cause breast cancer. They are permissive for further mutations that cause the disease. Women with the inherited BRCA1/2 mutation are born with the mutation—they inherit it from one of their parents. But they aren't born with breast cancer.

In many examples like this, there's a genetic vulnerability to cancer, but the cancer itself isn't inherited. The person merely inherits a predisposition; those who have the gene are more likely to develop cancer. What the BRCA1 and 2 genes do, probably, is interrupt the conversation taking place in your body to repair broken DNA. But not everyone who has the BRCA genes gets diagnosed with breast cancer. This is because, much in the way the body has several pathways leading to cancer, it also has several pathways to repair DNA. Keep in mind, too, that the majority of women who suffer from breast cancer have completely intact BRCA genes, so clearly there's more at play here than genomics.

Which brings me back to the notion of a system. How you arrive at an end point in a vast, complex system is somewhat irrelevant. It's caring for and protecting the system as a whole that can impact outcomes. More precisely, cancer is a symptom of the breaking down of the conversation that's going on within and between the cells. Somehow the cells are deciding to divide when they shouldn't, not telling each other to die, or telling each other to make blood vessels when they shouldn't, or telling each other lies. Somehow, all the regulation that is supposed to happen in this conversation is broken. When we see a whole bunch of cells starting to divide uncontrollably in an area, we call that cancer, and depending on the body part in which it happens, we'll call it lung cancer or brain cancer. But that's not actually what's wrong; that's a *symptom* of what's wrong.

The habit of describing cancer by body part came about from the combination of observations made on autopsies in France in the early 1700s and microscopic techniques developed in Germany in the mid-1850s. This hasn't changed since. It is utterly archaic that we call cancer by prostate, by breast, by muscle. It makes no sense, if you think about it. There used to be dozens of kinds of cancer, and now there are hundreds of kinds of cancer. In truth, there are millions of kinds of cancer. The average cancer has more than one hundred mutations in coding genes when it's first diagnosed, and I don't think there's any way to really comprehend or model that. The number of mutations shoots up exponentially as a cancer patient is treated with drugs such as chemotherapy, which inherently causes more mutations. One of the hallmarks of cancer is unstable DNA, so when chemotherapy drugs bind to DNA, they can cause cancer just as radiation can cause cancer by mutating the genome. This helps explain why survivors of breast cancer, for instance, can suffer from leukemia later in life due to the chemotherapy they received to cure their breast cancer. They made a trade of one illness for another but gained more years of quality life in the interim.

Tumors themselves should be considered organs; they are as much a part of our system as our liver, heart, and lungs. Cancer is a failure of the system, simple as that. To channel Tolstoy, happy families are all alike, but unhappy families are each unhappy in their own special way; and happy bodies are kind of all alike, but when they break down, they all break down in their own special ways.

We misunderstand cancer by making it a noun. I like to tell people that cancer isn't so much something that you "get" or "have" as it's something that the body *does*. Instead of saying, "You know, my house has water," we say, "My plumbing is leaking." Instead of saying, "Somebody has cancer," we should say, "They are cancering." We're probably cancering all the time, and our body is checking this problem in various ways to make sure that we're not cancering out of control. What keeps cancer under control is a conversation that is happening between your cells, and the language of that conversation is contained in your *proteins*.

Protein Power

We tend to think of proteins in terms of diet and nutrition; they are one of the three principal constituents of food (alongside fats and carbohydrates) that are known as macronutrients important to our health. But there's much more to the definition of proteins. They are essential parts of our bodies, and they participate in virtually every process within cells, including how cells talk to one another and orchestrate biological events that feed cycles of health or illness. The study of proteins is now a burgeoning new field called proteomics, and at the core of this exciting branch of research is the exploration of how proteins create the language of our bodies—and the language of health. Proteomics will allow us to listen in on that cellular conversation, which will lead to much better ways to treat cancer, as well as any other ailment or disorder.

Our DNA is static, but our proteins are dynamic. They change in your body every minute, depending on what's going on internally. I can't tell from looking at your DNA if you've just had a glass of wine, how well you slept last night, when you last had a meal, or if you are under a lot of stress. But your proteins, on the other hand, will tell that story. They will reveal information about you that you cannot find elsewhere in your body. Through proteomics, I can start to look at the "state" of your body because I'm looking at what you ate, what certain drugs you could be taking are doing to your body, how a long workout has affected you, etc. It's that twenty-thousand-foot view that allows me to look at the whole picture, at a moment in time, which DNA alone cannot provide.

Galileo's Genius

In chapter 5, I'll be taking you on a tour of proteomics and reveal where we are in this powerful new field. I have no doubt that this will change the future of medicine, as well as the future of our health. When it comes to a breakdown in the system that results in things such as cancer, autoimmune disease such as rheumatoid arthritis and fibromyalgia, or even unexplained chronic pain and nerve disorders, having a grasp of how proteins interact and change in the system could mean the difference between an endless battle to poorly manage a chronic disease and a real treatment that can end suffering. The idea that you should be able to take a pill, and it should magically fix the manifestations of a disease—a systems disease, a failure of the system—is quite remarkable. As I've noted, this approach is usually possible where you have an invader that doesn't belong and you take a pill that poisons that particular invader. Likewise, in a few cases where you're just missing one component to health, you can take a pill that provides the missing ingredient.

It's human nature to want to find magic bullets in medicine, but they happen once in a blue moon, and we may already have had all of our blue-moon moments. We haven't found many new pills lately that really cure diseases. This is why the pharmaceutical industry is somewhat broken right now; it has run out of low-hanging fruit, a magical chemical that cures a disease. I don't think we're likely to find a lot of more of those; it seems like a waste of time, money, and resources to keep looking for these magic bullets. We need a different approach—a new model.

The good news is that if we start to model the body as a complex system, which means controlling it without necessarily understanding every fundamental component, we might be able to actually get somewhere. We may never come to understand what maladies such as cancer actually are until we begin to view the body through a lens that can honor and appreciate its intricate, interconnected nature that begs to be controlled before it can be truly appreciated. Later in the book we'll see how proteomics helps us create this new model and begin to explore the body in ways we've never done before. But until proteomics becomes a mature and established area of clinical medicine through which all of us can benefit, we need to change how we think about health and, at least psychologically, recognize the body from a systemic standpoint.

We owe much of our understanding of the night's sky to a similar train of thought. In the early parts of the seventeenth century, Galileo would go out every night and map the stars in the sky. After a while, he had the map figured out and could peer into the sky on any given night and know what to expect; he'd know where the stars would be. But did Galileo know what a star even was? Not a chance. Neither did anyone else who'd been admiring these luminous patterns in the sky since ancient times. It would take science hundreds of years to figure that out. Galileo's genius resided not in his ability to understand the universe, but in his capacity to surrender that need to know so he could make progress in other areas of cosmology.

If I had to summarize it in a sentence, I could say that the biography of the human body is a biography of a system like no other. We may think we have a handle on certain aspects of it that deem it healthy or not, such as high or low cholesterol and ideal body weight, but these often lead to categorical and often uncompromising interpretations. Or, to put this another way, we may choose to take a B-complex vitamin to improve our energy and boost metabolism, but there could be a compromise elsewhere in the system as a result. What's "good" for one thing might not be for another. And "good genes," such as no history of cancer in our family, can sometimes betray us.

Cancer inspires fear not only because it's synonymous with a long, painful, and grievous affliction that rarely has a cure, but also because it's so stealthy, artful, unfathomable, and inherently baffling. Naturally, we don't like things that we cannot comprehend well or control. Perhaps that's why it can be equally as hard to grasp that the body is a complicated, and often mysterious, being. We don't want to admit that it's perplexing beyond modern comprehension, and that we may never be able to fully understand this body of ours the way we can understand English or how to ride a bicycle. Misunderstanding and ignorance beget fear. Still, the irony here is that if we have the courage to embrace ourselves as complex beings that are inexplicable in a lot of ways, and treat ourselves as such, we may move faster and closer to gaining that control we so desperately seek. We may also expel the fear that diminishes our quality of life.

Health Rule

We may never understand illnesses such as cancer. In fact, we may never cure cancer, which is why prevention is key. It's important to approach your health in general from a place of *lack of understanding*. Honor the body and its relationship to disease as a complex emergent system that you may never fully comprehend. Diseases such as cancer, heart disease, diabetes, autoimmune disorders, and neurodegenerative diseases reflect breakdowns in that system. Cancer, for instance, isn't something the body "has" or "gets"; it's something that the body *does*.

2

A Pound of Cure

*The Simple Ways to Measure Your Health Today and
Accept Trade-offs in Designing Your Health for Tomorrow*

It's easy to be swayed by general words of wisdom on health. Take a multivitamin. Eat more vegetables; maybe try juicing to save time. Consider a statin if you've got high cholesterol. Lower your risk for cardiovascular disease and cancer with daily baby aspirin. Get more vitamin D through supplements. Choose foods high in antioxidants. These all seem like pretty healthy notes of advice. But are they right for you?

In the upcoming chapters, I'll help you to answer that question, because many of these commonly held perceptions are just that—*perceptions*. I'm going to bust a few of these ideas and show you a different way of considering what's good for you or not. For now, however, let's revisit the notion of looking at the state of the whole body because I need you to understand a few more things before we get really personal. In this chapter, I'll delve deeper into the concept of appreciating the body as a system, help you gain an understanding of what it means to identify your *personal metrics*, then help you establish your baseline—the current state of your body—from which all preventive measures commence.

Accepting the Trade-offs

At this point I hope I've impressed upon you that a lot is going on in the body at any given moment. Yet we perform medicine in piecemeal—targeting one problem at a time. If you're diagnosed with pneumonia, then you'll receive a treatment specific for pneumonia and await your next health challenge. But what happens when you've got a system that's broken down in a way that cannot be explained by any single invader, bite, tick, virus, parasite, bacterium, etc? Then you've got a real problem on your hands because current methods in medicine don't know what to do with you. The proposed treatment will probably mess with other areas in your system in ways that we may or may not know about. Your doctor will tell you that that treatment is "safe and effective," but he's only talking in relation to that one condition, at that moment in time. He's not considering everything else that encapsulates you—especially in the long run—because a lot of that knowledge remains to be understood.

To illustrate what I mean, let's take statins as an example, the class of drugs that includes Lipitor and Crestor. Statins are among the most commonly prescribed drugs in medicine to improve blood cholesterol levels. They also brilliantly illustrate how certain external forces, in this case a drug, can have a measurable impact on the state of an entire biological system. Biochemically, statins are compounds that inhibit a liver enzyme that plays a central role in the production of cholesterol. These compounds can be derived synthetically or isolated from naturally occurring foods such as red yeast rice and

45

oyster mushrooms. Because it's believed that high cholesterol, especially of the LDL (low-density lipoprotein) kind, is a risk factor for heart disease, doctors like to dispense statins to people who cannot control their cholesterol through diet alone. But statins don't just affect cholesterol.

In one of the most important clinical trials in the long history of statin studies, researchers at Harvard showed in 2008 that taking statins can dramatically lower the risk of first-time heart attacks, strokes, and other artery problems in apparently healthy men over fifty and women over sixty years of age who *do not have high cholesterol*. We know now that the real underlying reason for cardiovascular events may not be all about cholesterol. Cholesterol could be the wrong indicator in many people, what we call a biomarker, and inflammation—a normal but sometimes overactive biological process—could be the better one.

Briefly, inflammation is a telltale sign that something isn't right in the body, that the body is encountering harmful stimuli, which can be any number of things from pathogens to damaged cells and irritants. To protect itself and try to remove the injurious stimuli, the body triggers inflammation, an elaborate response involving the vascular system, the immune system, and various cells within the injured tissue. The ultimate goal is to start healing, but when inflammation becomes chronic due to disease or prolonged stress, it can become destructive.

One of the ways we can measure inflammation in the body is by assessing levels of C-reactive protein (CRP), a protein whose levels increase when inflammation is present. This protein helped researchers figure out one of the major reasons why statins lower the risks of cardiovascular disease. The JUPITER study (*J*ustification for the *U*se of Statins in *P*rimary Prevention: An *I*ntervention *T*rial *E*valuating *R*osuvastatin) became the first of its kind designed to evaluate the effect of statin therapy on reducing heart attacks and strokes among people with normal LDL-cholesterol levels and elevated C-reactive protein levels. It confirmed that elevated CRP levels may indicate a risk of future heart attack up to eight years in advance, even if cholesterol levels are low.

Hence, statins may work their wonder by lowering inflammation—not cholesterol per se. So it should be no surprise that other studies have shown that when drugs effectively lower cholesterol but not inflammation, the frequency of heart disease remains unaffected. I'll be going into much greater detail about inflammation in a later chapter because it's a prominent subject in health circles today. Researchers are now discovering bridges between certain kinds of inflammation and our most pernicious degenerative diseases, including heart disease, Alzheimer's disease, cancer, autoimmune diseases, diabetes, and an accelerated aging process in general. Virtually all chronic conditions have been linked to chronic inflammation, which, put simply, creates an imbalance in your system that stimulates negative effects on your health.

All of this brings up a good point: it's quite arbitrary and unscrupulous to cherry-pick a variable such as cholesterol within a complicated system and ask, "Does this one variable get better with this pill?" and then say, "Okay, yes, it does." As a comparison, we may note that the motor's RPMs went up because we poured this goop into the engine, but is that really a good thing? Maybe the RPMs went up because it broke the regulator or because it clogged up the safety valve. Right now, when doctors test a drug, they are looking at one variable over a discrete period of time. They only discover potentially bad side effects in retrospective studies—looking back after people have been taking the drug for a long time, or by pooling several studies together. I hardly need to point out the obvious cliché that rings true here: hindsight is twenty-twenty. Wouldn't it be great to have perfect vision as you look at your future health? Wouldn't it be helpful to know what to do today to arrive at an ideal state of health? That's exactly what fields such as proteomics and other new technologies hope to facilitate. In the meantime, you still have an enormous number of tactical strategies that you can employ, which I'll describe shortly.

Most drugs have trade-offs. They shift the balance. There's a reason why you don't naturally produce statins. I don't think it's because nature didn't think of the idea. It's probably because statins have some pluses and minuses; what you're doing is rebalancing things, tipping your biology in a certain direction. I intentionally pick on statins because they are widely used for good reason and have had a great impact in cardiovascular medicine, lowering millions of people's risks for heart disease and stroke; they are the perfect example of a drug that changes the system in ways that, for most, are highly beneficial. The pros outweigh the cons, and later in this chapter you'll read that I'm a huge advocate for taking statins.

A particularly stark example of a trade-off can be seen in the recent trend among older men seeking the fountain of youth who inject themselves with human growth hormone. In 2009, Americans spent $1.35 billion on growth hormone treatments, filling 431,000 prescriptions, many at the request of people hoping to turn back their clocks. As the body ages, it doesn't produce growth hormone the way it did when it was younger and rapidly developing. Artificially using this hormone as an antiaging treatment might help you to build and maintain muscle mass more easily (the way you did when you were younger), but there's a big compromise.

In 2011, a study of an Ecuadorian population with a rare genetic mutation that prevents them from responding to human growth hormone found they almost never get cancer or diabetes. The discovery, published in the journal *Science Translational Medicine*, backs up earlier research showing that yeast, flies, and rodents live longer—in some species, as much as ten times longer—when they grow slowly. *Less* growth hormone—not more—may help prevent cancer and diabetes in old age. So, men who enjoy unnaturally larger muscles in their golden years due to growth hormone injections are accepting a much larger risk for cancer, diabetes, and probably other serious conditions. Research like this might lead to drugs that suppress growth hormone to prevent many diseases of aging, much the way statin drugs are used to lower cholesterol and prevent cardiac disease. The goal of such prevention wouldn't be to live longer, but to live disease-free for as long as possible.

We Are Not the Same as Before

This idea that we have to accept trade-offs in our lives when we take actionable steps to live the best life we can, or the life that we want, will always be part of our health strategy. However, we need to consider something else in our preventive tactics that most people haven't even thought about: weight. The population in the United States has radically changed in the past couple of decades just by observing changes in weight, as measured by body mass index (BMI). Twenty years ago, no state had an obesity rate above 15 percent; ten years ago, no state had an obesity rate above 24 percent. Today twelve states have obesity rates above 30 percent and thirty-eight states—two-thirds of all states—have obesity rates above 25 percent. Twenty years ago, the state with the highest combined obesity and overweight rate (Wisconsin) was 49 percent. Ten years ago, only

Globally, more than 1 billion adults are overweight, with at least 300 million of them obese. In the United States, only 33 percent of adults are at a healthy weight for their height. Obesity in adults and children, male and female, has doubled over the past forty years, with the biggest increase seen since 1980. Obesity and being overweight pose a major risk for chronic diseases, including type 2 diabetes, cardiovascular disease, hypertension and stroke, and certain forms of cancer. In fact, it's estimated that every third person born in 2000 will have type 2 diabetes as an adult.

two states (Alabama and Mississippi) had a combined rate above 60 percent. Now the lowest rate is 54.8 percent (D.C.), and forty-four states are above 60 percent.

When you look at the world data, it's similar to that of the United States. BMI is growing at an alarming rate. More than two-thirds of Japanese have a normal BMI, whereas fewer than half of the populations in Canada, Spain, and Australia have a normal BMI. In Great Britain, New Zealand, and the United States, roughly a third of the population is normal, and two-thirds are over the BMI limit for what's considered a normal, healthy weight.

It may not seem obvious to you, but these statistics demonstrate that our overall system today is remarkably different from what it was just a few generations ago. So the diseases we have today, which reflect patterns in the system over the last several decades, are going to change substantially over the next decade or so based on extraordinary shifts such as these, as will response to treatments. Studies done ten or twenty years ago may have little relevance today as a result. Local systems—"microsystems"—can exist as well, much in the way microclimates exist within a larger geographic area. The obesity rates in the South are much higher than those in such states as Montana and Oregon. Studies performed on those who live in Louisiana won't necessarily mean anything to people who live in Colorado, the only state holding strong with less than 20 percent of its population obese; that may have changed, however, by the time you read this. These reflect two entirely different systems existing within our population.

Ethnic factors can also be at play when we consider the results of studies. Obesity rates aside, microsystems can exist for other reasons, the most prominent of which is based on genetic risks shared within a geographic area. A community dominated by Ashkenazi Jews, for instance, will carry a different set of health risks from one that's predominantly Asian or African-American. When we read or analyze studies, such forces can often be grossly underestimated.

For example, studies carried out at the renowned Mayo Clinic in Rochester, Minnesota, may not have much significance to people who live in other regions of the country, say Newark, New Jersey, or New Orleans, Louisiana.

The reason for this has everything to do with demographics and the genetics of ethnicity. The Rochester community is heavily populated with German and Norwegian Americans who tend to marry and procreate within their community, thus maintaining a steady gene pool. Hence, their ancestry's genetics will be vastly different from that of a homogenous community elsewhere. The meaning of studies performed will be different depending on the group studied, even when the rigors of the scientific method are employed to generate a "randomized" group of participants. So the next time you read an eye-popping headline about a health-related study revealing something "new" (especially those that tend to be alarmist), look behind that headline to see where the study was done and who participated in it. Does it reflect you and your genomic ancestry? You just might find that you can ignore those findings, as they won't apply to you and your library of personal metrics.

Which brings me to the core question: what is a *personal metric*?

Defining Your Personal Metrics

In simplest terms, a personal metric is data point, rule, standard, or detail that says something about your health. Your weight, for instance, would be a personal metric. Your need to go to bed at exactly 10:00 p.m. to feel good the next day is a personal metric. From a broader perspective you can also look at metrics as a set of habits or customs you subscribe to that affect your health—that either enhance or detract from the state of body that you aim to achieve. In this manner, there could be healthy metrics and unhealthy metrics, but I say this with caution.

I'm hesitant to use those words *healthy* and *unhealthy* because these terms can be confusing. They are not necessarily polar opposites, despite the common perception of these designations. What's "healthy" for one person may not be for someone else. Moreover, these terms tend to morph into absolute labels on habits, foods, and drinks. Just as the words *good* and *bad* get thrown around like unconditional and categorical descriptors, the use of *healthy* and *unhealthy* lacks context in most cases. The context boils down to what your metric for "health" is. Most people, for instance, would say that a doughnut is not "healthy" (or "good"), but it's not fair to say a doughnut is "unhealthy" (or "bad") from a purely technical standpoint. If your metric for health entails the occasional indulgence in high-fat, sugary treats, then certainly a doughnut could be deemed "healthy." But if your metric for health shuns all foods made with saturated fats and refined sugar, then the doughnut probably won't live up to your standards for what's considered healthy. As I stated in the introduction, I'm not here to tell you what's healthy or unhealthy for you in absolute terms. I want to inspire you to create your own metrics and learn how to be your own advocate for your well-being.

When establishing your personal code of health, you'll have a unique set of health challenges to address, risks to bear, physiological advantages or disadvantages, and physical responses or side effects to drugs to consider. Health itself becomes a system—a system of checks and balances that you can attempt to control using all the knowledge that you have at any given time. This won't be an arbitrary practice because in the future you'll also have a way to test out what certain habits do to your system. You'll be able to spend a week ramping up your intake of lycopene, for example, and see what that does to your blood profile; then spend another week or so avoiding lycopene and compare that blood profile with the previous one. The secret to your health will entail a concert of habits that has an overall impact on your system and that favors health. You'll also be able to measure your system constantly using high-tech devices so you can continue to fine-tune and drive your body closer to the ideal picture of health.

Now it's time to get personal. I'm not expecting you to run out today and execute all of the ideas below. I want you to have this itemized list to keep for whenever you choose to address these matters. It would be unwise of me, as a physician, to not give at least some specific details on the practical and highly accessible ways in which you can measure the current state of your body. None of the recommendations outlined below requires a specialist or exorbitant amount of money. Much of the following is likely covered by your health plan; some of the tests mentioned can be obtained at pharmacies that offer walk-in clinics. Above all, this information aims to empower you with the road map you need to take charge of your health.

Be Your Own Doctor First

You typically visit your doctor once a year, if that. In this annual exam, he or she takes your vital signs, listens to your heart and lungs, may draw some blood for testing, has you pee in a cup, conducts some surface inspections, addresses any gender-specific tests to check breasts, uterus, testicles, etc., and asks a few easy questions, one of which will be *Do you have any specific concerns or complaints?*

If you don't have any serious issues, you breathe a sigh of relief and go about your merry way until next year, or at least until you get sick. Your doctor sees you at one specific time during the year. He won't necessarily know that your blood pressure spikes every afternoon unless you happen to be in the doctor's exam room when this happens, and he probably won't know to ask about your multiple trips to the bathroom in the middle of the night or your nagging lower-back pain, which you've accepted as a part of aging. Medicine is the art of observation and interpretation, which are skills that are not learned in a book. Until medicine becomes more of a science with the advancement of technologies, you have to find someone who practices this art very well. It matters who your doctor is and how you collaborate with him as a team on your health's playing field. Similarly, there's an art to knowing when to intervene. You and your doctor must have knowledge to make important decisions when they arise. The goal is to treat appropriately and avoid over-treating. Thankfully, modern medicine is moving away from the traditional "doctor knows best" paternalistic mode of medical decision making, in which health-care providers make key decisions for their patients. This type of decision making is slowing giving way to "informed choice" or "shared decision making," in which you make the final decision based on your goals, values, and tolerance for risk. Of course, informed choice demands that you be thoroughly knowledgeable about your health status and treatment options, which is what you'll achieve with the help of this book. Your doctor will also have to show signs of competence and act like a team player.

I implore you to ask your doctor, *How do you stay current?* Ideally, you want someone who stays up-to-date with the latest literature and technology. Asking this question isn't a threat. If your doctor is good, she will take it as a compliment. I find that people are overly worried about angering their doctor, which is a shame. It may be human nature to not want to upset somebody, especially somebody we view as in a position of power, but this is your health we're talking about. Playing nice won't result in you being treated better or your disease being diagnosed sooner. Much to the contrary, playing too nice and not challenging your doctors when they need to be challenged can leave you in the dust—literally.

You'll also want to find a doctor who helps you to make decisions based on your value system, which, as I just discussed, is key to making informed decisions. If you don't believe in undergoing surgery for back pain, for instance, because it has little guarantee of eradicating your pain given your unique condition, you'll want to explore other remedies that coincide with your values. Most decisions made in medicine today are based on someone's values, so be sure that your opinions and convictions are respected. There's rarely a "right" decision for any stage in disease. There's one for you, but there's no single "right" decision. The right decision for you will be the one you and your doctor arrive at together, whether that entails drugs, surgery, or a combination thereof.

Your goal is not to be friends with your doctor. It's a partnership, not a friendship. This is the person in whom you put faith to guide your life. Those are very different priorities, which most people don't comprehend. If you cannot tell your doctor anything, find another doctor.

Doctors like these are not hard to find. First and foremost, the information you bring to the office is what will make the difference in your doctor's capacity to serve you best. Though it may sound obvious, I want to make it clear that your health is in many ways up to you. If you frame the questions correctly and have your data with you, you can get what you want out of the conversation. So, with this in mind, I'll give you some tips about measuring your own health, collecting that data, and knowing how to talk to your doctor about any problems. Once you have your baseline established, you'll know how to consider certain habits, and in some cases medicines, to help you recalibrate your body toward health.

Establish Your Baseline

Just as your spouse or friends can't always definitively "know" what you want for your birthday without your specifically telling them, a doctor will only know as much about your medical history and any current issues that you're experiencing as you're willing to verbalize or reveal. There is no oracle for health when you show up for an examination. The knowledge *you* carry is more essential than your doctor's knowledge. Unfortunately, the economics of twenty-first-century medicine means that more and more physicians spend less and less time with patients. It's up to you to maximize that time.

Start by making a comprehensive list of things to bring up in your visit *before you step foot in the waiting room.* Do this exercise in the comfort of your home and use the checklist on pages 15 through 18 to perform a mini self-exam. This is step one in establishing your baseline. It's a rough way of sketching out and defining your current "state." It helps to keep a health journal for a time, during which you really pay attention to yourself and repeatedly fill out that questionnaire. See if you can relate your answers to last month or last year. What has changed? What has remained the same?

Bring a comprehensive list of all the medications (over-the-counter and/or prescription), vitamins, and supplements that you take, as well as their dosages and the frequency you take them. When in doubt about what to include, such as the Tylenol PM that you take on Sunday nights, include it! Make copies of any labels of supplements that have more than one ingredient. Any tests that your doctor wants to perform could be affected by the supplements you take, so speak up. Saw palmetto, for instance, can lower the value of PSA (prostate-specific antigen), which is a protein produced by the cells of the prostate gland in men. The PSA test measures the level of PSA in the blood, in hopes of detecting elevated levels that can signal prostate cancer. What's more, because PSA is controlled by testosterone, many times it's important to get testosterone levels checked simultaneously. If your testosterone is low, you'll have a different cutoff number for PSA; your doctor will look at your clinical situation differently than if you're producing a normal amount of testosterone and show low levels of PSA.

A doctor's visit is not the time to be shy and withhold information. Go in with a game plan, as if you're planning to ask for a raise from your boss. This means you show up with a list of your problems, questions, and everything that you want to get out of the checkup. Be honest and forthright. Your doctor will not judge you.

Don't wait to see if something gets worse before your next visit. If you have a little backache when you bend over, start talking about it today. You are your own barometer, and you have to keep the catalog of your own symptoms. Don't assume your doctor is going to ask you every possible question to arrive at every potential solution to your concerns now and in the future. Every sign and symptom you experience should be recorded and discussed. You want to ward off troubles before they anchor themselves. When you present this full report, you and your doctor can start to look for manifestations of certain diseases, as most are preventable or can easily be headed off before they become severe. I marvel at how some people pay attention to every detail of a stock they purchase but not to themselves. Why not? We want quick fixes, I know. We get overloaded with information. We can easily feel overwhelmed by our obligations and commitments in life such that we feel the need to trust someone else for our health decisions, such as our doctor. But I'm here to tell you, this won't keep you on the best path to health.

I also recommend that you bring a friend or family member with you when visit the doctor. It creates more accountability; you also have another set of ears. Many of us aren't in an ideal frame of mind when we're in the doctor's office, especially when something is wrong, so having someone else there can make the whole visit more bearable—and memorable. Alternatively, bring a way to record what you hear. Many smartphones today have a recording feature, or you can download an application to do so.

Now, let's move on to the more nitty-gritty details of what to request at your next visit so you can fully establish your baseline metrics in numbers. Again, this is just a basic outline to consider as a starting point. Your doctor may already have a recommended, and more comprehensive, list of items he or she will review during an annual checkup, so don't fret if this seems limited. I can't possibly cover every option that should be available to you based on your unique circumstances, so consider the following list as a general map for you overall "checkup" landscape. Have your doctor run the following tests, all of which can be obtained through a simple blood draw:

- *Fasting lipid profile:* This is a group of tests that are often ordered together to determine risk of coronary heart disease; they include your cholesterol and triglyceride numbers. You have to fast for about twelve hours prior to the test, but you can drink water.
- *Levels of high-sensitivity C-reactive protein:* As previously indicated, this is a biomarker of inflammation, which can point to your risk for cardiovascular trouble, among other things, if your levels are high.
- *Comprehensive metabolic panel (CMP):* This is a frequently ordered panel of tests that gives your doctor important information about the current status of your kidneys, liver, and electrolyte and acid/base balance as well as all of your blood sugar and blood proteins.
- *Complete blood cell count (CBC):* This is one of the most commonly ordered blood tests, which is the measure of the concentration of white blood cells, red blood cells, and platelets in the blood. The size of your red cells can be a good indicator of nutritional deficiencies. You want this number, called the mean corpuscular volume, or MCV, to be between 85 and 95 fl. You also want to see that your red cells come in all different sizes, which shows cells at different stages of their life span.
- *Thyroid stimulating hormone (TSH) test:* Your thyroid is your master metabolism hormone. If it's out of balance, guess what? So is your whole system. An underperforming thyroid (hypothyroidism) is one of the most underdiagnosed conditions in America, yet it's incredibly common—especially in women. It's believed that

20 percent of all women have a "lazy" thyroid, but only half of women get diagnosed. Unfortunately, no single symptom or test can properly diagnose hypothyroidism. To arrive at a trustworthy diagnosis, you'll also need to look at your symptoms. These can include weight gain, fatigue, constipation, hair loss, and even shortened eyebrows, as one of your thyroid's functions is to regulate how quickly your cells replenish themselves. When your levels of thyroid hormone drop below normal, the effect can be seen in almost every cell in your body, including hair follicles. To fix a thyroid problem, you'll also need to look at the whole picture—all the things that make up your lifestyle. (A rarer condition called hyperthyroidism happens when the thyroid goes into overdrive, producing too much thyroid hormone. This also has negative effects on the body, triggering heart and bone problems among other things.)

- *Hemoglobin A1C:* To understand what a hemoglobin A1C is, think in the following simple terms: Sugar sticks to things, and when it's around for a long time, it gets harder and harder to remove. In the body, sugar also sticks, particularly to proteins. The red blood cells that circulate in the body live for about a hundred days before they die, and when sugar sticks to these cells, it gives doctors an idea of how much sugar has been around for the preceding three months. In most labs, the normal range is 4 to 5.9 percent. In poorly controlled diabetes, it's 8 percent or above, and in well-controlled patients it's less than 7 percent. The benefit of measuring hemoglobin A1C is that it gives a more reasonable view of what's happening over time (about three months), and the value does not bounce as much as finger-stick blood-sugar measurements. While there are no guidelines for using hemoglobin A1C as a screening tool, it gives a physician a good idea that someone is diabetic if the value is elevated. It's one of the few tools doctors can use to look at an "average" in you that you cannot fib. Diabetes can just happen. It's not just about being overweight, so if you suddenly develop this disease for whatever reason, you don't want to miss that.

Although your doctor will test your vitals, you need to remember that she is only testing these metrics at one particular moment in time. She won't have running averages for your numbers over the past six months. While it's common for many of us to keep track of our weight throughout the year, we might also want to track other metrics—and should—if we're at risk for certain things. You can easily track your temperature and blood pressure using kits you can buy at your local pharmacy. You may want to check your blood pressure at different times of the day two or three days a week to see what kind of fluctuations you're getting. Make a spreadsheet and start to record the numbers at certain intervals throughout the day. Add notes to indicate what's going on when you take the test, such as that you've just had a relaxing glass of wine or just got off a troubling phone call that made you tense. Bring that spreadsheet with you to your doctor.

Men only: When you get a PSA test, have your testosterone levels checked as well. Testosterone controls levels of PSA, so your body's production of testosterone will affect your parameters for "high" versus "low" levels of PSA. What's considered high for one person might not be the case for another person. Also, abstain from sexual activity and bicycle riding for several days prior to the test. While these activities don't affect the PSA level of everyone, they can negatively influence results and cause undue stress if you're told to repeat the test.

Depending on your age and unique risk factors, you and your doctor will explore other tests. Mammograms, colonoscopies, Pap smears, PSA and testosterone tests, and so on should all be considered in relation to your situation. If close blood relatives have suffered from certain types of cancer at a relatively young age, then you should discuss being tested for that cancer sooner than current recommendations for the general public dictate. If you eat a lot of fish, especially swordfish and tuna, a blood mercury test might also be helpful.

Ask about vaccines and other preventive measures you can take that are relevant to you, your age, and your risk profile. The shingles vaccine, for instance, might be something you want to consider if you're sixty years of age or older. Do what you can to keep abreast of well-documented studies on preventive measures you can take for known risk factors. Until proven otherwise, most people should be taking statins after the age of forty, and especially those with elevated cholesterol and/or elevated C-reactive protein—both of which are risk factors for heart attack and stroke. If you're over forty and bear any risk factors for cardiovascular disease, I encourage you to figure out with your doctor why you *shouldn't* be on a statin.

I reiterate: this is when supplying your doctor with all the information you've got about your history and lifestyle is invaluable for making decisions and choosing the best course of health care for you. But please don't leave everything in the hands of your doctor. Ask questions. Understand the whys, hows, and whats. The more you know, the more you'll be able to stick with your doctor's recommendations, and the more you'll understand his or her answers, as well as the parameters given.

One more tip. Before you leave the doctor's office, be sure to ask:

- What should I focus on this year?
- How can I get copies of my results?
- What tests are being performed on me?

- Do I have baselines to refer to in case things go wrong?
- Which vaccines should I consider now and in the future?
- Given my history and profile (age, risk factors, etc.), did any studies come out this year that are relevant to me?

This last point should not be taken lightly. While I was writing this book a new study surfaced that went largely unnoticed by the mainstream public. It reported on some unexpected positive effects that taking a baby aspirin can have on reducing one's chances of dying from many common forms of cancer. We've known for some time that a baby aspirin a day can help prevent blood clots and stave off a heart attack or stroke, but now we have another benefit to attribute to this miracle pill for people nearing their fifties and above. In this new report, stemming from eight long-term studies including some twenty-five thousand patients, British researchers found that a small, seventy-five-milligram dose of aspirin taken daily for at least five years reduces risk of dying from common cancers roughly 10 to 60 percent. Here are some of the findings, published by the *Lancet*:

- After five years of daily aspirin, death due to gastrointestinal cancers decreased by 54 percent.
- After twenty years, death due to prostate cancer decreased by 10 percent.
- After twenty years, death due to lung cancer decreased by 30 percent (among those with cancers typically seen in nonsmokers).
- After twenty years, death due to colorectal cancer decreased by 40 percent.
- After twenty years, death due to esophageal cancer decreased by 60 percent.

Caution: these findings don't necessarily mean you should start a daily aspirin regimen; it can still be responsible for some complications, such as bleeding, that have historically kept it from being recommended for daily consumption for everyone. But the report demonstrates major new benefits that have not previously been factored into guideline recommendations. Prior guidelines have rightly cautioned that in healthy middle-aged people, the small risk of bleeding on aspirin partly offsets the benefit from prevention of strokes and heart attacks. But the reductions in deaths due to several common cancers may now shift this balance for millions.

Does the balance tip the scales in favor of your taking a daily baby aspirin? That's a question for you to answer with your doctor. While the study didn't find any difference in the results between men and women, the age of the patients affected the findings significantly; older patients benefited a lot more from daily aspirin than younger ones, and the ideal candidates for a daily dose of aspirin are probably those nearing their fifties. Researchers will continue testing to explore these promising initial results, but in the meantime it's exciting to know that we might already have an effective cancer-battling drug on hand in our medicine cabinets.

Aspirin has been around as an analgesic for aches and pains for more than a hundred years. Its active chemical ingredient, acetylsalicylic acid, is from a class of drugs that have been extracted from plants ever since Hippocrates left historical records describing the use of powder made from the bark and leaves of the willow tree to help alleviate headaches and fevers. Aspirin has broad effects on the body, which is why this wonder drug has the capacity to address so many ills—from tinkering with the pathways that result in the sensation of pain to preventing heart attacks by keeping blood clots from forming and reducing the risk of cancer likely through a variety of mechanisms. Aspirin is, above all, a powerful anti-inflammatory, which might explain why it's such a panacea of sorts.

Just as you should talk to your doctor about whether you should be taking aspirin, you need to do the same with all of your prescriptions. Every time you visit with your doctor, make a clear follow-up plan. If you are sent home with prescriptions, whether they entail drugs or not, ask how you will know what works and what doesn't. How do you find the treatment that does work? Which seasonal factors should be noted? If you don't visit your doctor more than once a year, you need a game plan that covers you for the whole year. If you're in the doctor's office in May, for instance, you won't be able to get a flu shot. So you need to keep an open line of communication year-round to take into consideration the variables that naturally occur monthly and seasonally.

Remember, there's a lot of trial and error in my business. We don't have the technology yet to precisely predict what medicine you'll respond to or which one will work best. Make sure that when you take something, it works! If you regularly take pain medication as a habit but feel no pain, why are you still taking it? Be your own regulator, and you will get closer to a regimen that meets your medical needs.

Is There an App for That?

I'll admit I'm a techie. I love gadgets. I'll also admit that I have an abnormal EKG (electrocardiograph, which measures the electrical activity of the heart). My T wave is inverted and I've accepted that this is how I was built. It's not terribly abnormal, but it's there. If I land in the hospital and cannot communicate for whatever reason, all my doctor has to do is download my EKG record on any computer by accessing my Apple MobileMe account, which is an online storage site that I subscribe to that allows me to safely keep information on the Internet. Today it's known as cloud storage. (Assuming that my cell phone will work in the hospital, I can just download it myself on my iPhone and show to a physician.)

We use our phones and computers today for just about everything. With one exception: storing our medical records and keeping our health metrics in check. I've got all of my baseline records stored in my mobile cloud so it's always accessible to me. I've also given my wife all of my passwords so she can access this same file when and if that becomes necessary. I believe that everyone needs a partner in health care. This person can be a spouse, sibling, parent, friend, or neighbor. Pick someone. Give that person full access to all of the places where you keep your medical data.

What if you don't have your medical records nicely organized in digital files? Don't worry, most of us fail to keep digital records. Most of us still have the bulk of our files stashed in hard copy written in barely legible handwriting, collecting dust in our doctor's archaic filing system. I implore you to request copies of all your files from all your doctors. Spend a Saturday afternoon creating digital copies of them using a scanner. You can also keep them on a USB key chain that you take everywhere. I realize that this could be asking a lot from you. But it's just a few hours of work that can benefit you over and over for the rest of your life. We are all unique and have abnormalities. It's nothing to be ashamed of. But what makes us different can make us a challenge for doctors who don't know anything about us if we haplessly, unexpectedly land in their emergency room or office someday. Having your entire medical record on file to hand over just might save your life.

Every day new digital applications emerge that can help us to track our health and even our attempts to live an active, healthy life. I can't even begin to list them all here because an astounding number are available, and by the time you read this a whole new generation of useful software programs will surely have hit the market. You can track, calculate, plan, and research just about anything health-related these days and personalize that info for yourself. Sleep apps can help you analyze your sleep patterns, heart apps can help you track your stress level (some can allegedly help with your emotions), and some apps can notify you of the foods in your geographical area that are in season and provide information on local farmers' markets.

Pretty soon we'll be able to wear little devices that can clue us in to our body's dynamics all day long. Not that we all may want to wear such gadgets 24–7, but these could be incredibly powerful tools for creating and maintaining baseline numbers, and in some cases for training ourselves to know when we could benefit from some "tweaking." It's hard to take yourself from a raging bull in terms of stress back down to a calm, cool cucumber, but if your body could somehow tell you that you're entering a danger zone, this could motivate you to make effective changes to reduce your stress.

Tools are critical to our success in so many areas in our life— e-mail and cell phones to communicate, Internet to research, cars to get to where we are going, etc. Why would we think that we don't need such help with our health efforts? The tools are already at our fingertips. Using them will propagate those incentives we need. Make it a goal to study yourself consistently and keep charts. Listen to your body and remember, only you know your body best. There's no way your doctor can be inside your body or your head. You have the ability to follow the trends that relate to you. Find them. Start living your healthy life today. And as you'll see in the next chapter, knowing where you came from can further help you to *plan* your future health.

Health Rule

Don't put blind faith and trust in your doctor. Be your own doctor first. Use the combination of the questionnaire on page 15 and the guidelines in this chapter to empower yourself with the information you need to define your personal prescription for health. When working with your doctor on your protocol, view the relationship as a partnership—not a friendship. Also, don't entrust your doctor with storing all of your medical information. Request copies of your data and store it in a readily accessible place online.

3

Go Back to the Future

Why It Pays to Know Your History—and How to Get It

How many of our grandparents died "of old age"? In many cases familial relationships may not be ideal, and conversations loaded with questions about health can be difficult to broach. As a result, we can find ourselves filling out health-history questionnaires in our doctor's waiting room pondering questions that we should know the answers to, such as, does mom have soaring cholesterol? What killed Uncle Earl? Is there any diabetes or cancer in the family? Perhaps you don't realize that the hunched back of Grandma and her sisters could foreshadow your osteoporosis. Or maybe Dad never mentioned that in his forties he survived a mild heart attack, the same affliction that killed his own father at an early age. Patterns of familial illness can predict someone's brewing health risks, so gaps in this history can be problematic.

Most families don't ask questions of their family members, especially the elders. But the surest way to escape more invasive tests is simply to muster the strength to ask the tough questions. I'm assuming, of course, that you have access to at least some blood relatives or old health records and were not an orphan or part of a blind adoption. Family history is one of the most underused but extremely powerful tools to understanding your health. In 2010, one study by the Cleveland Clinic concluded that learning about your family tree is the best tool to predict genetic cancer risks. Such a tool is free, even if it entails a discomfort factor, or perhaps a long-distance phone call. All it costs is a little time questioning your relatives. Good family health trees are rare; a government survey estimated less than a third of families have one, and time-crunched doctors seldom push their patients to remedy that.

If querying Grandpa or your great-aunt over the phone sounds daunting, then make it a goal to initiate the conversation at your next holiday gathering. Reunions and even funerals can also make for ideal places. The US surgeon general operates a free website—https://familyhistory.hhs.gov—that will help you to create a family health history and share it electronically with relatives and your doctor. Don't dismiss one side of the family, especially if you're a woman who knows less about your paternal relatives than those from your mother's side, which is common. The threat of breast or ovarian cancer can lurk on either side of the family.

Because genes seldom render our destiny, a family health tree should also reflect shared environmental or lifestyle factors that can further affect an inherited risk. Who smoked? Who was overweight? What other forces were working on those in the family who died prematurely? The answers to these questions can be enlightening on many levels and can lead to better personal care. Once you exhaust the limits of this kind of rough detective work, you may want to consider taking it to the next level: genetic screening.

Consider Genetic Testing

If you've spent any time watching the news or reading any kind of publications in the last decade, then you know that we've accomplished a huge undertaking that commenced in 1990: we've determined the sequence of nearly all the 3-billion-plus chemical building blocks that make up the human DNA code. I briefly introduced DNA in chapter 1, implying that it says less about you than you might think. But I haven't gone into full detail about how it works, what it really says about you, and how you can maximize its utility. Now let's step closer to this piece of information so you can understand it properly in the grand scheme of your health. I'll then cover some of the basics to modern genetic screening.

The genetic code, also known as the human genome, is found in virtually all of the trillions of cells in the human body and provides the instructions for how human beings operate. This code is strung together into twenty-three "volumes of information" called chromosomes. We each possess two sets of each chromosome, with one set inherited from each parent. Chromosomes are composed of strands of DNA, which in turn are made up of tens of thousands of genes. DNA's well-known double-helix structure is connected by rungs of approximately 3 billion base pairs, represented by four chemical bases, or nucleotides, known most commonly by the letters A (adenine), G (guanine), C (cytosine), and T (thymine). These nucleotides are key structural elements for the genes that individually or in combination determine everything from a person's hair color to their predisposition for Parkinson's disease.

After thirteen years of work, the project was declared complete two years ahead of schedule in 2003, coinciding with the fiftieth anniversary of Francis Crick and James Watson's Nobel Prize–winning discovery of the DNA double helix. Certain sequences of these building blocks make up genes, just like certain sequences of letters create words. Now the race is on to decipher the meaning encoded by these 20,000 to 25,000 genes, which are essentially the molecular remote controls to our body's functionality. Genes are what determine many aspects of yourself, such as whether you have blue or brown eyes and the likelihood that you will suffer from obesity or Alzheimer's disease. A *genome*, by definition, is the entire set of hereditary instructions for building, running, and maintaining an organism, and passing life on to the next generation. Each of Earth's species has its own distinctive genome: the dog genome, the cat genome, the genomes of the rose, rabbit, cold virus, broccoli, *Escherichia coli*, and so on. The genome contains all of the information necessary to produce a specific organism. Genomes belong to species, but they also belong to individuals. With the exception of identical twins and other clones, every person has a unique genome, as does every deer, oak tree, and eagle. Genomes are different between individuals as well as species.

Among the groundbreaking findings uncovered by the Human Genome Project was that approximately 99.9 percent of DNA sequences are similar across the human population. Single nucleotide polymorphisms (SNPs, typically pronounced "snips") represent variations in DNA sequences and occur every one hundred to three hundred bases along the 3-billion-base genome. SNPs are alterations in the set of genetic instructions that are thought to provide the genetic markers for our response to disease, environmental factors, and drugs. For example, an A instead of a G on a particular gene may indicate a trait for male-pattern baldness. Other variations in nucleotide sequences may provide a marker for celiac disease, cystic fibrosis, or asthma. It's important to realize that these DNA differences do not cause the disease, but they are a marker of the relative risk of the disease. Since the completion of the Human Genome Project, hundreds of studies have been published that describe the associations between SNPs and hundreds of specific diseases, traits, and conditions. As you can imagine, these studies have opened the door for the personal genomics industry by providing a platform by which DNA, obtained through a simple saliva sample, can reveal your individual genetic map.

As a cofounder of a company that performs genetic screening, I'm obviously a big proponent of this technology, which takes a broad look at these DNA variations to offer clues to your risk for certain ailments. Even though DNA sequencing may only give you a general list of your "ingredients" without telling you exactly how those ingredients mix and interact in your body, it provides an important foundation—the more you know about your overall ingredient list, the better you'll be able to make decisions about your health. This type of screening can give you the heads-up on what to look out for when evolution is no longer taking care of you as you age. It's not a diagnostic test; it won't tell you if you have lupus or cancer, for instance. Genetic testing shows genetic predisposition to common conditions, so that prevention measures may be taken or early diagnosis may be made. The degree of genetic risk you inherit is related, in part, to how many risk markers you have residing at each SNP—none, one, or two. Just because you may have one or two risk markers does not mean that you will definitely develop a given health condition, but it can raise your risk, especially if other lifestyle or environmental risk factors are present. In many respects this is similar to other tests we regularly use in medicine. If an individual has an elevated cholesterol level, for example, we consider that person at a higher risk for cardiovascular disease and consider preventive measures.

The concept behind locating genetic markers, these SNPs, is fairly straightforward. Take thousands of people with a medical condition, and thousands of similar people who do not have that condition. Compare their DNA and identify places where one variation of a marker is much more common among the affected people than the healthy people. Your own genetic markers are then compared with the data reported by researchers in scientific journals, the results of which can then be converted to a more accessible scale: your estimated lifetime risk of having that condition. These SNPs may not actually cause the condition, but we know they are either part of or close to genes that increase the risk of that condition and are therefore used as markers of increased predisposition to that condition. If you have no known genetic risk markers for a condition, it doesn't guarantee that you won't get it, but it does mean that your risk is lower than that of people with those particular risk markers.

Keep in mind that these health conditions have many causes, genetic and environmental, some of which are not yet known. Currently, we can look at genetic risk profiles for about forty conditions, from aneurysms to multiple sclerosis to stomach cancer. All of this data can be determined from saliva. No blood drawing is necessary, as there is enough DNA in saliva to be amplified and studied. Some genetic tests, such as those that check for the BRCA gene mutations—the high-risk indicators for breast and ovarian cancer—can require a blood drawing. It depends on who is performing the test and how they prefer to obtain your DNA. Tests can also be done on hair,

Here's a sampling of conditions for which we currently have genetic tests for risk profiles:

Cancers: breast, colon, lung, prostate, stomach, melanoma

Autoimmune: Graves' disease, lupus, psoriasis, rheumatoid arthritis

Vascular: abdominal aneurysm, aortic aneurysm, brain aneurysm, deep-vein thrombosis

Vision: macular degeneration, glaucoma

Neurologic: Alzheimer's disease, multiple sclerosis, restless legs syndrome

Cardiac: atrial fibrillation, heart attack

Gastrointestinal: Crohn's, celiac disease

Endocrine: type 2 diabetes, obesity

Joint: osteoarthritis

Other: sarcoidosis, hemochromatosis

Pharmacogenomics: dose and response to a group of drugs that span several diseases skin, and amniotic fluid. Most pregnant women today are offered genetic testing and genetic counseling to identify their baby's vulnerabilities to inherited diseases and disorders.

A small handful of companies have emerged to conduct genetic testing. At my company, Navigenics, our mission is to empower people with genetic insights to help motivate them to improve their health. I'm a firm believer in the power of this technology, which will continue to have more utility as we add more medical conditions to the existing list and learn about new associations between DNA variants and certain illnesses, and the pharmacogenomics data is expanded. Pharmacogenomics, as you'll read about shortly, is another burgeoning new branch of pharmacology that deals with the influence of genetic variation on drug response.

When people receive a report from Navigenics, which is designed to be reader-friendly to the average individual who doesn't have a medical degree, they obtain access to ongoing information relevant to them through the Web and based on new research. They also learn how they can modify their current behavior to reduce their risk of various conditions that they may be more susceptible to based on the research, the dose of and response to certain drugs, and what they should tell their doctor. Even though these reports are easy to read and digest, the data can be overwhelming and comprehensive, so we strongly encourage people to speak candidly with their physician so they can understand the meaning of it all and how they should proceed. Everyone who undergoes the test is also encouraged to discuss the results with the Navigenics team of genetic counselors specifically trained to deal with the issues that this predisposition testing brings up. My hope is that information like this can motivate people to change their behaviors so that a healthier life awaits them.

The other benefit to genetic testing, and one that will rapidly expand its precision with the advent of proteomics, is the kind of custom-tailoring we can do in drug therapy. We can now conduct what's called a pharmacogenomics analysis to analyze your DNA for genetic markers that are known to affect how your body might process certain pharmaceutical drugs. In some cases, your genetic code can indicate whether you are likely to experience severe side effects with a particular drug, and in other cases whether the drug is likely to be effective for you, or how to dose the drug perfectly for you. By knowing how you are likely to respond to certain medications, you and your doctor can work together to make medication choices tailored for you.

It all comes down to incentives. I can tell you that you have a 30 percent chance of becoming obese based on the general population, which is probably meaningless to you. But if I could tell you that your risk of becoming obese in your lifetime is 60 to 80 percent based on your genetics, this would likely mean something, wouldn't it? That might be enough to inspire you to pay more attention to the lifestyle habits that factor into your weight. That might be enough to motivate you in ways you never thought possible to control your waistline. That's the power genetic testing can have on individuals. Another way to look at it: if you knew that your personal risk for having a heart attack in your life was 90 percent, you'd probably do everything you could to treat your heart well. Hearing another umbrella statistic such as "heart disease is the leading killer in our country" has little impact, if any. But learning that your genetic profile puts you in a higher-than-average risk group for suffering from a heart attack speaks much louder than general statistics.

This kind of information ultimately allows you to consider the personal trade-offs that you might have to accept. For example, if you know that you possess a higher risk of developing heart disease, then drinking a glass of wine a day could be a good thing to make part of your health protocol, assuming you enjoy drinking. We've known for some time now that moderate alcohol intake, especially from red wine, can reduce one's risk for heart disease but potentially increase one's risk for breast cancer. This is the trade-off, and together with your doctor you can weigh those pros and cons to create a personalized health plan.

Based on all of the above information, would I suggest that you get your genetic profile today? As with most of my suggestions in this book, this one is up to you. If you are uncertain of your health history and have no other way to gather the information, then by all means consider participating in one of these services. Most Flexible Spending Accounts and Health Savings Accounts will reimburse you for the out-of-pocket expense if your health plan won't cover it. For any diseases that are more or less deterministic—a known mutation makes it highly probably that you will develop the affliction—then I encourage you to find out and take the appropriate steps to avert or delay that fate. Examples of these rare genetic disorders include BRCA 1 and 2 (breast/ovarian cancer), Tay-Sachs, and Huntington's disease. Whatever testing you do undergo, plan to participate in genetic counseling, as well. This will not only help you to fully comprehend your risk profile, but also help you to manage any mixed emotions that surface. This is also a great training ground for understanding lab reports.

My personal Navigenics profile turned up some interesting results. I have an above-average risk for cardiovascular disease, even though my lipid prolife was normal with a total cholesterol level of less than 200 (anything less than 200 is considered good to normal). Based on my risk profile, my doctor and I decided that I'd start a regular regimen of Crestor, one of the statins; and my kids took it upon themselves to keep me away from french fries. Ironically, that same year I began taking a statin, the JUPITER study came out to show the benefits of statins for not just lowering cholesterol but for also lowering inflammation in the body. Now the research is on to study people with low markers of inflammation and low cholesterol to see what statins can do. What else might they affect?

My profile also pointed to a slightly lower-than-average risk for colon cancer, but after questioning family members, I learned that a close relative had colon cancer. I then chose to undergo a colonoscopy at age forty-three, rather than waiting for my fiftieth birthday as recommended by national standards. My family history indicated too high of a risk for me to have waited. The genetic testing, together with a good family history, changed my personal view on health. I ended up having a polyp removed. Polyps are abnormal growths of tissue that can become cancerous. Could my polyp have turned into cancer? Who knows? But why should I have waited for that to happen? Being proactive, I intervened and kept my healthy state on track. This is exactly what you should be doing, with the doctor you choose to guide you continuously down a healthy path. The key is a good family history together with the genetic testing. Unfortunately, family histories are difficult and many times misleading. Many diseases were considered bad words in previous generations, and accurate information about family medical issues can be difficult to obtain.

Will you be able to handle the results should the tests find something? That's a question we all ask ourselves. What if, for example, it's discovered that you carry the [APOE] e4 variant of the APOE gene, a variant that has been found to increase the risk of developing Alzheimer's disease? Few of us can predict how we will respond to any negative news related to our health, or even the risk to our future health. But here's an encouraging fact: when researchers from Boston University School of Medicine studied children of parents with Alzheimer's disease who were informed that they carried the e4 variant of the APOE gene, the researchers learned that the short-term distress of having a positive result might not be so damaging.

The report, which was published in the *New England Journal of Medicine* in 2009, came out of the REVEAL Study (Risk Evaluation and Education for Alzheimer's Disease) and was the first randomized trial to disclose to participants whether they carried the gene variant. As expected, people who were stressed out about the test beforehand and who tested negative were relieved. But those who had to endure a positive result only experienced a temporary blip in their emotions. The psychological impact wasn't nearly as terrible as one would have guessed, and it disappeared quickly. The lead author on the study, Robert C. Green, a professor of neurology, genetics, and epidemiology at Boston University as well as a fellow in genetics at Harvard Medical School, stated, "Participants who learned they were [APOE] e4 positive and were therefore at increased risk for Alzheimer's disease showed no more anxiety, depression, or test-related distress than those who did not learn their genotype." Rather, Green claimed what I've long believed, saying, "Learning genetic risk information can be a positive and empowering experience for some people, even when the disease is frightening and the genetic information has no clear medical benefit."

When it comes to deciding whether to obtain certain genetic information about yourself, I think it's less of a question of "Would I want to know?" and more a question of "How will I take action today?" if you do learn that you're at a higher risk for certain ailments. The adage rings true: information is power. If you don't know, you can't know how to live your best life to safeguard the future you. I was skeptical myself at first. I didn't think that my results would affect or change me. But I still remember the Friday night I came home and my results were available over the Internet. I was a bit scared to see what I'd find, and what my future held, but when I saw myself on the computer screen, I felt a profound sense of awe. I was actually seeing me, and it indeed changed me right there on the spot. I modified how I ate, how I exercised, how I lived. The experience also changed my entire family because obviously my results had implications for my children. As a family we began to make improvements to our lifestyle choices. I can't think of a better impetus to change than having a personal peek at your own set of genes and what they potentially portend for you. It's empowering, not terrifying.

My Personal Genetic Profile

Condition	Your percentile[1]	Your estimated lifetime risk[2]	Average lifetime risk[3]
Abdominal aneurysm	75%–100%	3.9%	3.1%
Atrial fibrillation	0%–59%	22%	26%
Brain aneurysm	75%–100%	0.80%	0.64%
Celiac disease	10%–12%	0.01%	0.06%
Colon cancer	30%–33%	5%	6%
Crohn's disease	40%–42%	0.36%	0.58%
Deep vein thrombosis	82%–87%	3.3%	3.4%
Diabetes, type 2	22%–24%	19%	25%
Glaucoma	43%–79%	0.78%	1.1%
Graves' disease	11%–36%	0.39%	0.55%
Heart attack	71%–87%	46%	42%
Hemochromatosis, HFE-related	0%–57%	extremely low risk / no risk markers present (non-carrier)	N/A
Lactose intolerance	95%–100%	high risk	N/A
Lung cancer	33%–80%	8%	8%
Lupus	32%–37%	0.01%	0.03%
Macular degeneration	39%–48%	1.3%	3.1%
Melanoma	72%–92%	5%	3.7%
Multiple sclerosis	37%–57%	0.17%	0.30%
Obesity	55%–85%	36%	34%
Osteoarthritis	11%–18%	26%	40%
Prostate cancer	46%–48%	16%	17%
Psoriasis	20%–23%	2.8%	4.0%
Restless legs syndrome	56%–72%	4.3%	4.0%
Rheumatoid arthritis	10%–17%	0.88%	1.6%
Sarcoidosis	21%–69%	0.61%	0.70%
Stomach cancer, diffuse	0%–13%	0.65%	2.4%

[1]**Your percentile:** This information allows you to see how you compare to other people. Compared to a sample population, your SNP-based risk for the condition is within the given range of percentiles.

[2]**Your estimated lifetime risk:** Your risk of this condition over the course of your lifetime. For some conditions, estimated lifetime risk numbers are not available. In these cases, we indicate whether you are at increased risk for the condition.

[3]**Average lifetime risk:** The average person's risk of this condition over the course of their lifetime, depending on gender. For some conditions, such as hemochromatosis and lactose intolerance, average lifetime risk estimates are not available.

Note: Black boxes indicate either that your overall risk is greater than 25 percent or your risk is more than 20 percent above average for that condition.

Source: Navigenics.

Above is my personal genetic profile, which I am sharing with you exactly as the report reads (footnotes are obviously speaking to me). This was a wakeup call to me. My risk of cardiovascular disease is real, and I took action.

Nature vs. Nurture

As a prelude to the next chapter, take a look at the following charts that display how much genetics or, conversely, environmental factors play in various disorders and diseases. It's quite thought-provoking to actually absorb these percentages and think about how much we can affect the outcomes in our health lives. Some of these illnesses would seem to be controlled largely by genetics, but remember, the environment can play both direct and indirect roles in our health risks. Environment, which entails a mesh of overlapping factors from diet and exercise to exposure to toxins and stress, can ultimately affect the genes that you've inherited for good or bad. The genetic side of the equation here represents inherited risk factors—they are not necessarily causal genes to the ailments. So, for example, if you look at obesity, 33 percent of this disease is attributed to environmental influences; and 67 percent is attributed to inherited markers on particular genes that can increase risk but don't necessarily cause obesity per se. If your DNA profile puts you at a higher risk of developing obesity, that doesn't mean it's your fate. You can take control of the environmental side of the equation and reduce your overall lifetime risk by a lot.

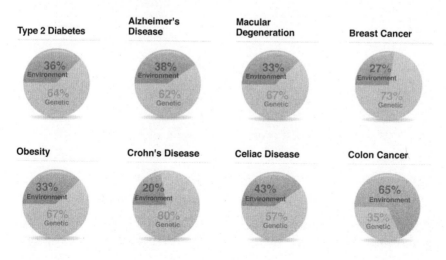

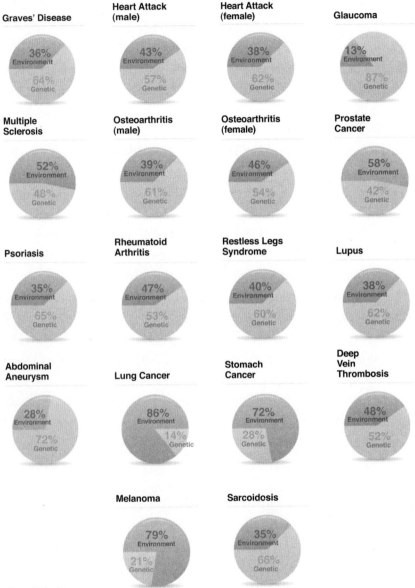

Source: Navigenics.

This is an important distinction because, as I noted earlier, far too many people adopt fatalistic views when it comes to their DNA and how it translates to their health. As we'll see in this next chapter, the difference in the environment can mean everything. And by *environment* here, I'm referring not only to the obvious ingredients that make up that word, but also the environment on a cellular, systemic level that affects how drugs work and whether you respond to treatments in pursuit of health.

Health Rule

Face the facts: Know your genetic risk factors for disease by getting a DNA screening test, but also understand that DNA governs probabilities—not destinies. There is so much you can do to shift your fate and live longer and better than what your DNA seemingly dictates.

4

Rotten Eggs and Cute Chicks

How Environmental Impacts Can Be Huge Where We Least Expect Them, and Insignificant Where We Most Expect Them

We just saw how much nature (DNA) or nurture (the environment) factors into an assortment of common diseases today. Obviously, we cannot change genetics, but we can change our environment to affect genetics. There's no better way to illustrate this concept than to share with you what I call the Egg Concept. I was originally told this by one of the greatest cancer researchers and thinkers in biology at Johns Hopkins, Don Coffey, Ph.D.

If you take an egg and let it sit at room temperature for a few weeks, guess what you get: a spoiled, rotten egg. But if you take that same egg and, instead of letting it spoil on a counter for three weeks, you subject it to a cozy 99.5 degrees Fahrenheit and rotate it three times a day, the outcome will be totally different: a chirping baby chick. (Note: the rotations must be an odd number; go figure. For the record, a "century egg" or "hundred-year-old egg" is something entirely different, as it's created using a unique process of preserving an egg in a mixture of clay, ash, salt, lime, and rice hulls for several weeks or months. That one can create a century egg by carefully exposing it to certain ingredients adds more credence to the argument: environment can mean everything.)

This simple experiment demonstrates the profound effect that environmental nuances can have, as gravity and temperature turn chaos to order. Similarly, little changes in our system can have dramatic overall effects. But we're often not thinking about all the possible little changes that can happen under our radar and which can work against us or help us stay healthy.

In searching for a way to bring this into practical, human context, consider the studies that have been done on the effects that the uterine environment can play on a growing fetus—a developing egg that has been fertilized. Given the volume of research that has emerged in the last several decades on prenatal development, no one would argue this vulnerable period isn't the staging ground for both well-being and disease in later life. We know now that moms who put on too much weight can increase their child's risk for diabetes, that low birth weight can increase the chance for cardiovascular disease later in life, and that exposure to chemicals, including alcohol, can trigger defects. More recently, researchers have discovered that even the internal environment that a woman maintains *between* pregnancies can have an impact.

In early 2011, Columbia University researchers determined that the risk of an autism diagnosis in a second-born child rose more than threefold when the child was conceived within twelve months of the birth of the first baby. Second-born children conceived between twelve and twenty-three months after a first child was born had twice the risk of being diagnosed with autism compared to babies conceived a full three years after an older sibling was born. Whether it's a deficiency in nutrients or a change in biochemistry, something happens in that uterine environment following a pregnancy that can affect the next one. The finding lends credence to earlier research on other brain diseases, several of which found that shorter intervals between babies are associated with mental illnesses such as schizophrenia.

Autism may well be a disorder brought on by many colliding factors that include genes and the environment. This recent discovery at Columbia, however, makes a stunning case for environmental influences that may not have anything to do with underlying genetics, or which dominate the unique circumstances that result in this heartbreaking diagnosis for most parents. The World Health Organization recommends that for having healthy babies, women not attempt another pregnancy for twenty-four months following childbirth. This advice is rarely heeded in many parts of the world, first-world countries included.

Perhaps the greatest demonstration of the power that certain surroundings and conditions can have on a living creature is found in how some drugs work. As an example, let's consider one of the most fundamental clinical trials in cancer, which was published in the prestigious *New England Journal of Medicine* in February of 2009. The researchers, many of whom hailed from the University of Vienna, Austria, studied women who were premenopausal with breast cancer. This is a particularly nasty type of breast cancer. The women had what's called hormone-receptor-sensitive breast cancer, which meant that their tumors grew when exposed to the female sex hormone estrogen. Thus, standard treatment often entails antihormonal treatment to combat the cancer-feeding estrogen. After the surgical removal of their cancer, the researchers then randomly created two groups from the 1,803 women. Twice a year, half were given a placebo (a dummy injection) and antihormonal therapy, and the other half received antihormonal therapy and a drug called zoledronic acid, which builds bone. Marketed in the United States under the brand name Reclast and Zometa, zoledronic acid is used to treat the bone disease osteoporosis. The result?

Those who received the bone-builder experienced a reduction in their recurrence of the cancer by 36 percent. Here's the stunning part: this particular drug doesn't even touch the cancer. This case demonstrates that if you change the soil (breast cancer classically metastasizes to bone), the seed (the breast cancer cell) doesn't grow as well. The drug changed these women's systems, thereby having a marked effect on their cancer. Five years after diagnosis, more than 98 percent of these breast cancer patients were alive—and the other stunner is that this outcome was achieved without chemotherapy. How exactly was this possible? We don't know, which reiterates the need for more data to understand the human body's complex system. Other experiments soon followed showing that taking bisphosphonates for osteoporosis for more than a year is associated not only with a reduced risk for breast cancer but also a reduced risk for colorectal cancer. Clearly, multiple things are happening from a physiological standpoint as a result of a single drug's ability to effect multiple outcomes. Researchers have postulated that the bisphosphonates reduce cancer cells' ability to travel and stick to each other (and to bone); that bisphosphonates stimulate cancer-fighting T cells; that bisphosphonates inhibit the formation of blood vessels that grow and feed cancerous cells; and that bisphosphonates increase the effectiveness of other anticancer agents while triggering the programmed cell death that keeps the body's cells in balance. More data will also allow us to make the kinds of inferences that will lead to useful experiments like the one I just described.

Similarly to statins, with their diverse, system-wide effects on the body, bisphosphonates are proving to have many potential uses other than preserving and building bone, and having anticancer effects. It's recently been shown that people who take bisphosphonates are gaining an extra five years of life. When a group of Australian clinical researchers first ferreted out these results from the world's longest-running large-scale study of osteoporotic fractures in men and women, they thought there had been an error, or that something had been overlooked. For example, an obvious factor could have been that the participants were people who had gone out of their way to get medical attention and do something about their condition, a trait that would predispose them to being healthier and living longer. But comparison of the results with those of similar health-aware participants taking vitamin D and calcium or women on hormone therapy confirmed that the results were not skewed by that factor. The drug was changing people's systems in more ways than one and tipping the scales in favor of health.

Thinking outside the box, these researchers speculated that one of the reasons could be that bone acts as a repository for toxic heavy metals such as lead and cadmium. As people get older they lose bone, and this is accompanied by a release of the toxic materials back into the body, which has a negative effect on health. Hence, by preventing bone loss, bisphosphonates prevent some of this toxic-metal release. Whether this is true will be determined by future research, but it proves one important fact that I've been detailing: a single drug can have an amalgam of effects, whether for good or bad. It can change the environment from which health or illness manifests. As with any drugs, the decision to take bisphosphonates should be made individually with your doctor. If given the choice, I'd take the extra five years of life assuming the drugs were right for me and my health metrics.

The Perils of a Petri Dish and the Promise of Observing Real People

Despite chemotherapy's being a widely used treatment for cancer, nobody has ever shown that most chemotherapy actually touches a cancer cell. It's never been proven. Researchers can perform all this elegant work in tissue-culture dishes—*if I expose a cell to this cancer drug, here's what happens*, and so on—but doses in those dishes are nowhere near the doses, nor the environment, that happen in the body. Thus I'm skeptical when claims are made about "anticancer" foods and nutrients. Sure, garlic and turmeric might assassinate tumors in the lab, but how does that work in a live body? The body is more complex and secretive than that. Certainly, consuming garlic and turmeric could be healthful, but we have to be careful about drawing hard and fast conclusions based on what's observed in a very controlled petri dish. Alcohol kills cancer cells in a petri dish, but not all alcoholics are cancer-free. Kerosene probably kills tumors in the lab, too, but we're not about to add that to our daily regimens anytime soon. We do, however, know that a toxin of a relatively less deadly sort works in cancer patients.

Chemotherapy clearly benefits cancer patients, yet frequently we can't explain why. In addition to the cases I gave above, I'll give you one more example that hit home for me because I ended up being a part of this experiment. It underscored the role environment can play in the growth and control of a tumor. It also demonstrated the extent to which experimentation—from petri dishes to people—can have unbelievable and unexplainable outcomes.

In 2001, I was part of the formation of a new nonprofit created to research new treatments for brain cancer, called Accelerate Brain Cancer Cure (ABC²). ABC² had been founded by the families of Dan and Steve Case, as Dan had just been diagnosed with a deadly form of brain cancer called glioblastoma multiforme. Steve Case is best known as the cofounder and former chief executive officer and chairman of America Online; his brother died of this rare cancer at age forty-four in 2002. In 2004, I received a call from Henry Friedman, one of the great neuro-oncologists in the country, based at Duke University. At a dinner he had met Virginia Stark-Vance, a solo practitioner in Dallas and Fort Worth, Texas, who was seeking advice for a patient, who also had the same type of advanced brain cancer, and chemotherapy hadn't helped. People with that condition have a life expectancy in single-digit weeks. This patient, whom we'll call Lucy, had done some homework and read in the *New York Times* about targeting cancers of all kinds with a drug that inhibits new blood vessels from developing and carrying vital nutrients to a tumor so it can thrive and grow. Seems sensible, but this drug, Avastin (the generic name is bevacizumab), had been approved only for colon cancer at the time—not brain cancer. The article in the *Times* was enough to convince Lucy and her husband that they needed to get their hands on Avastin; frankly, they had nothing to lose. But Stark-Vance had a few concerns, the chief one being that Avastin could cause bleeding in the brain. That had happened in one of the earliest clinical trials when a twenty-nine-year-old woman, whose liver cancer had spread to her brain, collapsed from a hemorrhage while riding her bicycle. Nevertheless, Stark-Vance decided to take the risk and green-light the Avastin treatment upon gaining Friedman's encouragement.

The call from Henry describing Lucy's initial results, as well as those from several other patients, revealed a very different outcome. I sensed a palpable excitement in his voice as he reported several impressive responses in which the cancer seemed to go away or not progress. This doesn't happen much in advanced brain cancer.

Like many others taking Avastin, Lucy had plunged into the unknown, without the assurance of a clinical trial studying whether the drug worked for her type of cancer. Doctors such as Stark-Vance and myself are free to prescribe Avastin, or any other drug on the market, for unapproved uses, at our discretion (it's called "off-label" use). As much as 75 percent of cancer drug use is of this off-label variety. Some of us doctors admit that with patients dying, we simply cannot wait for airtight evidence. What was really "off" about this experiment was that Avastin couldn't even get past the blood-brain barrier—it was too big of a molecule. So how could it do anything for a brain tumor? It turns out that this drug effectively changed the pressure in the brain; it changed the environment in which the tumor could grow. (For the curious, the drug is a well-documented ingredient in changing the pressure of organs.) Lucy's tumor required high pressure to grow, and Avastin—even though it couldn't touch the tumor itself—could lower the surrounding pressure in the brain and slow the tumor's proliferation. Here again we have a case of changing the soil so the seed doesn't grow so easily. When Duke University performed a clinical trial using Avastin on brain tumor patients like Lucy, 63 percent responded favorably to the drug— the patients experienced a dramatic delay in the progression of their disease and gained more time to live. In May of 2009, the FDA approved Avastin for the treatment of patients with brain tumors like Lucy's that have progressed despite other therapies.

In addition to illustrating the environmental impact on the progression, and certainly instigation, of cancer, another phenomenon that cases like this highlight is the serendipity often found in my field. Doctors such as myself arrive at solutions through plain old trial and error, and therefore we can't always explain how things work. I can't always tell you why a certain drug works or how it works other than to say I have seen results proving that it does. I also can't always give you a straight answer as to which course of therapy might work for you.

The story of Lance Armstrong's recovery is no more exemplary than other such stories that define my field. It's also emblematic of this new way of thinking and approaching disease. Scientists still have no idea why the combination of drugs Lance received cured his cancer. His intrepid, can-do nature doesn't solely explain his marvelous recovery. In fact, doctors—myself included—don't actually know why these drugs kill cancer cells at all! Those who are familiar with his story or who read his poignant memoir, *It's Not About the Bike: My Journey Back to Life*, know that in the fall of 1996, Lance was told to go home and spend time with his family once it was determined that his testicular cancer had spread to his brain, lungs, and abdomen. All of his doctors agreed that death was looming, and that further treatments were worthless, bordering on the absurd. But he would not accept this bleak fate, and like so many other patients desperate for a miracle cure, Lance hunted down a last-ditch option through relentless personal research, finding himself in Indianapolis entering an unusual three-month clinical trial led by Lawrence Einhorn and Craig Nichols. (Mind you, this was before the Internet took off and before Lance could conduct his hunt easily through the power of research engines such as Google; his relentless and focused nature certainly served him well here.) These two curious physicians were attempting to treat cancer patients with high doses of a drug derived from platinum, the same precious metal found in expensive jewelry and wedding bands. And it worked. Thirty months after receiving the drug, Lance had escaped the statistics in the halls of medicine and gone on to defy the odds on another playing field when he won his first of seven consecutive Tour de France cycling races.

Many of the drugs I use today, which clearly work, have arrived at their current utility by accident. The platinum-based drug that was so critical in the treatment of Lance's cancer had originally been shown to have anticancer effects in the early 1970s. Barnett Rosenberg was studying the impact of electromagnetic radiation on bacterial cell growth using platinum electrodes. He saw that the bacteria underwent substantial changes in structure when exposed to the platinum derivative created in his experiment (this derivative was cis-platinum—the same drug Lance received).

My point is not to come down on our having to accept serendipity in medicine and trial and error that can be frustrating. To the contrary, we should have more faith in experimental treatments and be willing to take those risks that can lead us to greater volumes of data. Being fierce advocates for our health requires that we view studies with critical eyes and, at the same time, be willing to push our boundaries when it comes to understanding how the body works—especially when it does things that seemingly defy previous logic or comprehension.

The medical field is so good at reporting negatives. We also need to report positives. Any time a patient of mine has a serious negative reaction to a drug, I am required to report this to the FDA. But I never have to report the positive! We desperately need the collection of data regarding treatments and outcomes for many diseases so we can learn from our mistakes as well as from our individual successes.

Two additional lessons can be culled from Lance's experience. First, he missed the early-warning signs that could have helped him avoid most of his cancer battle altogether. When it comes to ailments such as cancer, prevention and early detection are the keys to survival. Second, rather than accepting defeat or the common clinical wisdom about his particular affliction at the time, Lance educated himself and became his own advocate to find a personalized approach—albeit a desperate one—that had the potential to change his health outcome. It saved his life.

Shades of Gray

My field in particular is a breathtaking spectrum of gray shades. Most people don't understand that if your cancer is four centimeters in diameter and you come back four months down the road and the cancer is now six centimeters, we call that resistant—your cancer is resistant to the drug I was giving you and getting much worse. But maybe it would have been twelve centimeters in diameter without the therapeutic interventions taken. Using current technology, there's no way to know for sure. Most of the studies on resistant cancers use these metrics, which makes the results hard to understand. Defining true "resistance" becomes impossible. The medical field has evolved to be a binary field—yes versus no. But in reality it's a giant shade of gray that we cannot qualify because we don't have all the necessary data. We're only looking at two points, "before" and "after" in many cases, and cannot grasp the whole picture. Unfortunately, our only metric for success in my field is shrinking a tumor. Slowing down its growth isn't usually accepted as success, but I think it should be. After all, it can extend people's lives.

Case in point: In 2003, the drug gefitinib (brand name Iressa), which had been shown to interfere with the proliferation of lung cancer, became the center of attention when it reached the third phase of a clinical trial. Patients who were on the drug showed improvements in symptoms, *but their tumors didn't shrink*. This outcome alone, coupled with the lack of a placebo group in the study, tainted the study's positive results. Luckily, the following year a similar drug called erlotinib (brand name Tarceva) was put to the test using a placebo group, and again researchers showed that the drug helped most people with lung cancer live longer even though their tumors didn't shrink. This time the scientists could tell that the drug was prolonging the lives of patients, since their placebo counterparts died much sooner. Ideally, it'd be nice to conduct more of these types of studies without having to sacrifice a placebo group.

I'll give you one more example that epitomizes the complexity of the human body. If I prescribe to women with breast cancer a drug called paclitaxel (brand name Taxol) every three weeks, which is the standard today, about 40 percent of them with metastatic cancer will have a great response to that drug. A "great response" here means that those women will show a 50 percent shrinkage in their tumor. The cancer will then come back—the cancer "recurs," and the patient "relapses"—and I'll give those same women paclitaxel every week at a different dosage instead of every three weeks. Thirty percent will respond. The cancer will return for a third tour, and I'll administer paclitaxel over ninety-six hours by continuous infusion, and 20 or 30 percent will respond. I cannot tell you that the drug is working by the same mechanism in all three scenarios. It's not. We have no idea of the mechanism. Chemotherapy may be changing the environment in a way that disrupts that complex body system, just as building bone disrupted those women's systems and reduced their breast cancer's recurrence. Just as Lance's platinum-based drug reversed his fate.

In short, all of our systems are changing—constantly. They're dynamic, and they're a lot more dynamic than what we can do with test tubes and tissue cultures. My hope is that a new generation of therapies will address changes in the system, effectively shifting the body's environment in ways that can move it toward a healthier state. It's quite possible that we already have all the drugs we need to treat the vast majority of diseases—even the ones that entail a breakdown of the system and aren't caused by an invader. We just don't know how to use this library of drugs (method), how much to use (dosage), and when (schedule). New techniques for collecting health data in the future will hopefully inform this idea. Given all the examples I've described of how certain drugs work by simply changing the body's, or a certain organ's, environment, we have to wonder, what other drugs that we already have available for illness X can work wonders on diseases Y and Z?

The idea that the environment—and, specifically, changes to the environment—can play a defining role in both the treatment and progression of disease also applies in the development of drugs in general. When people ask me why most cancer drug development in lab animals doesn't work or cannot easily be applied to solve human problems, I explain three chief reasons. First, tumors grow slowly in humans as compared to in lab animals, where we can grow tumors in two weeks that represent 20 to 30 percent of the animal's whole body size. That's a staggering growth rate. So if I take a drug and give it to a mouse, and the drug causes some nausea, causing the mouse to eat less food, that mouse's cancer will grow much slower. The tumor is starved as the cancer's source of nutrients is truncated, and the cancer likely needs lots of nutrients to grow, because it is dividing more frequently than normal cells. Is the drug really working or is it because the mouse eats less? There's no way to control for this in an animal lab experiment. The two "environments" of humans and lab animals are radically different.

Second, it's hard to compare human tumors with those in other animals. Human tumors tend to be unique, and when we try to replicate a human tumor in another animal, we cannot achieve the exact same characteristics to study and manipulate. And, as we've already seen, the environment is key to a tumor's growth, and mimicking the same environment in a lab animal as in a human body is challenging, if not impossible.

Finally, controlling for the way various drugs work in different living bodies also presents an insurmountable challenge. A cascade of events happens when I administer a drug to a human versus another animal, and that cascade will depend on individual factors including metabolism, dosage, time, and so on. Again, replicating the same exact drug testing in two separate bodies is difficult, and interpreting the results from those tests given the variables can be even more difficult.

Until we have better methods for looking at illness from a systematic viewpoint, we cannot presume to prevent, treat, and ultimately cure our nemeses that so shrewdly evade our attempts to understand them. The good news, however, is that I believe we're swiftly approaching a revolution in biomedical engineering that will force us to embrace a new model for examining the body as a complex system. This revolution will endow us with the data we desperately need to optimize our individual health.

The Macroview

When you started this chapter, you might have been led to believe that "environmental impact" would somehow relate to our outside environment, such as the role pollution, exposure to environmental toxins, and the like affect our system. I intentionally covered the more "microscopic" view before saying anything about the other end of the spectrum—the macroscopic perspective. It's common knowledge now that our world is not as clean as it used to be. City dwellers live with higher degrees of air pollution; artificial and genetically modified ingredients find their way into our foods and beverages; plastics that leach chemicals are in household goods and drinking bottles; sometimes we can't be sure what's in the water supply; and industrial chemicals are ubiquitous even if you don't live near a belching manufacturing plant.

These factors can certainly disrupt your system, not to mention the system that is our planet's environment, but we should be careful about making broad claims and assumptions that all changes to our environment are "bad" from a health standpoint. The way in which compounds frequently dubbed "bad" affect our system may not harm our overall health. Each of these compounds and factors needs to be studied individually. We cannot forget that since we've moved into cities, our life expectancy has gotten longer—despite all the issues with cities and mounting pollution. Some of this fact can be attributed to better health care, but we still shouldn't make generic statements until each of these changes is studied closely and understood. We simply need more data to make definitive conclusions—to know whether or not we're going to get a rotten egg or a cute chick.

Health Rule

We can't change genetics, but we can change our environment to affect genetics. This can be done in myriad ways both internally and externally to impact our bodies' systems—and how they function. We might already have all the drugs we need to prevent and cure all illnesses, but we don't know how to use them appropriately to create those environmental changes in our bodies to achieve this. Gathering that knowledge will entail a combination of efforts from research circles, but also from citizens like you and me as we take charge of our personal health care.

5

Two French Restaurants, One Without Butter

The Weakness in DNA and the Power in Proteins

If I were to ask you what's the difference between how many genes a human has and the number of genes a fruit fly possesses, you'd probably assume that number would be pretty large. Humans are, after all, physically so much bigger, and vastly more complicated (though we can't fly, we can do much more brainy tasks). But strangely, the number of human genes seems to be less than a factor of two greater than that of many much simpler organisms, such as the roundworm and the fruit fly. But we make up for this seemingly paltry level of equipment in how we utilize our genes. Human cells can produce several different proteins from a single gene, and the human proteome—the biological treasure chest of all the proteins that cells can create—is thought to be much larger than those of our less complex creature-neighbors on the planet. Current estimates put the number of different proteins in the body at close to 1 million. Therein lies an important fact: our body's makeup is not so much about our DNA as it is about our proteins and the environment in which they are created. Let me explain.

I've already pointed out that DNA governs probabilities more than it dictates destinies, but I still find that many people hold on to the belief that your genome is equivalent to your "blueprint"—it's the instructions your body follows to make you, well, *you*, and affects whether you have a heart attack at forty-two or smoke a pack a day until you're ninety-two, at which point your heart finally gives up. Unfortunately, the blueprint analogy is misleading. Blueprints typically indicate how everything is connected, and how the parts relate to each other. The genome has a digital readout, but the problem is that we as humans are analog—not digital. We have continuous variables all over the place inside our bodies. So even though we can find out that your genome reads "ATCD" in one particular region, the task of figuring out what exactly that means in the extraordinary dynamics of your human body, and how that sequence codes for proteins that have specialized functions in you, is an analog process. My work with Danny Hillis has taken this challenge to heart, as we try to understand disease from an entirely different perspective from DNA alone.

I first met Hillis in May of 2003. Former vice president Al Gore introduced us following a visit Gore made to my lab at Cedars-Sinai Medical Center in Los Angeles. Gore, endlessly on a mission to change health care, had launched a campaign called Bluesky to Blueprint following his tenure in the White House. While I was showing Gore my lab, I explained to him that in order to really understand what we were up against in the cancer realm, we needed more than just the tools provided by genomics and imaging. In other words, studying DNA sequences, X-rays, MRIs, and the like wasn't enough. These sources of information had value, but they lacked dimension and dynamism. I also told him that we needed a way to understand outcomes of disease—we needed to figure out a way to take a drop of blood from a person and identify proteins within that blood that were associated with disease. Moreover, we needed to take that same drop of blood and have a way of determining the "state of the body," including that individual's metabolism and whether he or she carried disease.

You'd think that we would already have this kind of technology in medicine, a special kind of "health-o-meter," but we don't. As I've already conveyed to you, we can measure certain finite things in blood, such as sodium content, red blood cell count, cholesterol, and so on, and I can perform various tests on you to identify signs of infection or illness, and I can even sequence your DNA. But none of this really tells me about the overall "state" of your body. Sure, I could draw some general conclusions about your health based on these specific findings, but none of it would necessarily be all that helpful in identifying your overall "health."

I know that I piqued Gore's interest that day with my excitement about what the world of proteins could offer, but I also know now that I had cornered myself. Gore detected that I was in over my head given the volume of data I was trying to mine, and he said point-blank: "You need an engineer. You gotta meet this guy from Disney."

I wasn't in the mood to meet Danny Hillis, a person whose name I kept hearing over and over in the beginning of 2003. At the time I wasn't quite sure what he could do for me, being adamant that I didn't need an engineer described as "fantastic," "creative," and a "big thinker." Hillis hailed from the world of computer engineering and had recently left Walt Disney Imagineering to start a think tank in the San Fernando Valley in Glendale. I didn't believe that an ex-Disney guy who pioneered the development of so-called parallel supercomputers could offer me anything in my biomedical bubble. I would later learn that Hillis was equally hesitant to team up with me, "another doctor."

I eventually surrendered and never looked back once I met Hillis in person. Descriptors such as *fantastic, creative,* and *big thinker* don't begin to do this visionary justice. We became instant collaborators, and for his every computer-engineering yin, I had my biomedical-engineering yang that promised the possibility of changing how we studied the body and collected data. We started interacting regularly to apply engineering principles to my study of proteins. Our work started to bear fruit, and a company, Applied Proteomics, as well as a large National Cancer Institute–funded academic collaboration were born.

I've learned a lot from Hillis through the years, and we laugh now when we reminisce about how we first linked up. He has an uncanny way of distilling complex themes in my world down to simple terms that not only help the average person understand, but also help to create a refreshing shift in perspective. As Hillis describes it, DNA is more of a list of parts than a comprehensive blueprint. In this manner, DNA is more similar to a list of ingredients in a restaurant. In fact, let's do an exercise that Danny described to me once and that will help you grasp where I'm going with this. Think of your favorite restaurant. Now pretend that you want to figure out the health of that restaurant. If you had a list of all the ingredients that the restaurant has in its kitchen, you might be able to tell some things about it. You could probably tell the difference between a French restaurant and a Chinese restaurant just by the list of ingredients. But you wouldn't necessarily be able to tell the difference between a great restaurant and a rotten restaurant, a healthy restaurant and a sick one. The human genome is a lot like that. You can tell the difference between a European and an Asian just by looking at their ingredients lists, but you probably can't tell a lot about their general health. You probably can't decipher anything about a lot of things, such as their personality, intelligence, social mores, and general habits, and whether they prefer chocolate or vanilla. Something else to consider: when you're sick, you're still carrying around the same DNA as when you were healthy. Still, what does this indicate about defects in the genome?

Let's go back to the restaurant analogy for a moment. If a French restaurant was using margarine instead of butter, that might be a problem (a "defect"), or if a restaurant had a lot of salt, you might suspect that it had a predisposition to use too much salt in its dishes (another "defect"). But to really know what was going on, you would need to taste the food. The list of ingredients isn't enough. The quality of the food depends on lots of details of how they get combined and processed—on the cooking. In the human body, this "cooking" is about how the body processes the DNA through its magical mix of creating proteins.

Where Darwin Got It Wrong in Our Understanding of DNA

Genetics has had its day in the limelight for good reason. For one, DNA is among the greatest theoretical triumphs of biology. It may even be the biggest success story in biology because it started as just a theory and was later confirmed to be correct, which hardly ever happens in the field. By contrast, this order of events happens all the time in physics. Before we could prove the existence of black holes, for instance, someone came up with a model—an equation more or less—that indicated that they were out there. And lo and behold, black holes were eventually "discovered." As I mentioned in the introduction, Murray Gell-Mann first predicted the existence of quarks by creating a model based on mathematics rather than observation.

This type of discovery, whereby an abstract theory precedes actual proof, or even a way of testing out a theory, almost never happens in biology. Biology is rife with dogma based on real-life observations rather than postulations. That is, with one relatively recent exception: the field of DNA and the genome. Genes were theoretically predicted by the abbot Gregor Johann Mendel in the nineteenth century, who gained posthumous fame as the father of genetics. Mendel, an Austrian Augustinian monk as well as a passionate gardener, bred peas in the garden at St. Thomas's Abbey and took note of the effects of crossing different strains of the common plant. He is often immortalized as a kindly old man who, while puttering around his brotherhood's garden as the resident farmer, somehow stumbled onto important genetic laws. In many ways, though, Mendel was ahead of his time—acting more like a twentieth-century biologist displaced into the wrong century.

By systematically breeding peas, Mendel demonstrated the transmission of characteristics in a predictable way by inherited "factors" that would later be called genes. Although not all the technical vocabulary was in place yet to define his observations, Mendel basically demonstrated how characteristics get passed on from one generation to the next, and that for each characteristic in an individual, each parent contributed to that characteristic. He further showed that genes could have variations, resulting in dominant and recessive traits. One of the more important facts that Mendel proved, which became his most fundamental principle, was that genes do not "blend" in the offspring; rather, each genetic character is produced by a pair of gene variants called alleles, and that alleles segregate during the formation of male and female sexual entities (i.e., pollen and ovule in the case of plants; sperm and egg in the case of animals such as us). Members of a pair of alleles may differ in their expression, with one dominant over the other; and the combination of alleles in the next generation is a matter of chance. To put this into more practical terms, when you cross a blue-eyed cat with a brown-eyed cat, you can get a combination of blue- and brown-eyed offspring depending on how the alleles mix, and whether or not that brown-eyed parent is passing on a recessive gene for blue eyes. The brown-eyed parent could carry the recessive allele for blue eyes, but it's masked by the allele for brown eyes, which is dominant.

Whether or not you understand the logistics of passing on genetic traits is somewhat beside the point. Mendel's developing principles would become the basis for the new field of genetics, but they still lacked the "it" factor—the common denominator to all these observations and formulating principles. Charles Darwin, the English natural historian and geologist who was off making his own observations at the same time that Mendel toiled in the garden, may have made a better name for himself as the nineteenth century's greatest biologist and the father of evolutionary biology. But Darwin didn't have a real grasp of the principles of inheritance the way Mendel did. In fact, most of Darwin's ideas about hereditary mechanisms were categorically wrong.

Darwin believed in the blending theory, that the "blood," or hereditary traits, of both parents came together in the offspring just as two colors of ink blend when mixed. But the blending theory didn't work for continuously graded traits such as height and weight. If it did, then offspring in every generation would always be less extreme than their parents for every trait. Over time, the world would be filled with a bunch of "averages," which clearly isn't the case. Darwin's sharpest critics called him on this flaw in his theory when he finally got around to publishing his ideas on natural selection. The critics were right to point out that natural selection does not work with blending inheritance because any variation will be blended away. But even in the face of criticism, Darwin failed to come up with an answer. He even began to backtrack, and in later editions of his seminal work, *On the Origin of Species*, his explanations reflected echoes of desperation and exasperation.

The irony of Darwin's struggle is that he came close to solving the mystery of the laws of inheritance. His thinking was on the right track when he began to do some experiments with snapdragons in an attempt to resolve this nagging puzzle once and for all. He observed how one trait in a snapdragon could be eclipsed by another in the offspring, an observation of genetic dominance. But Darwin never crystallized these observations in the way that Mendel did. While Darwin was working on his snapdragon experiment in England, Mendel was making scientific history. Though the two would never meet, they performed nearly identical experiments and witnessed almost exactly the same results. For Darwin's part in explaining the fundamentals of evolution, luckily he only needed to notice that offspring tend to "resemble their parents" and leave it at that. This was obviously sufficient enough to hoist his grand theory on natural selection and propose the concept of survival of the fittest. History has spoken, because most people can define Darwin's claim to fame, but not Mendel's.

By the beginning of the twentieth century, we still didn't have a clue as to exactly what was responsible for all these developing laws of inheritance. Mendel's work wasn't published until 1866 and went unnoticed and unappreciated until the turn of the century. It would take nearly another century from Mendel's publication for science to dig deeper, when James Watson and Francis Crick proposed the double helix, or spiral staircase, structure of the DNA molecule in 1953. In essence, Watson and Crick officially discovered DNA, changing the textbooks forever now that we had an image of what "the secret to life" actually looked like. Such a feat has an almost religious significance in biology. Suddenly, we had a seemingly tangible thing to help explain what makes us tick and how we are made at the molecular level. All of the observations made by researchers such as Mendel and Darwin, and proposed "factors," could now be traced to a single, underlying, and seemingly omnipotent molecule called deoxyribonucleic acid, or DNA.

As a society searching for a better understanding of ourselves, we hold a special reverence for DNA. We not only anticipated that DNA existed long before we had proof, but we even were bold enough to forecast that we would one day decode what DNA actually meant, and we checked that off our list of to-dos with sequencing. Once we knew how to work with DNA in the lab, the field of genetics exploded. In the early 1980s Kary Mullis figured out an elegant way to study genes with practical tools that most biologists already had at their fingertips. It didn't take much to perform experiments on DNA in those early days other than having the right chemicals to trigger the right reactions. In the most elementary sense, you simply heated a DNA-containing sample up and cooled it down a few times, then you poured it in some Jell-O, ran a battery across it, and out came a readout of the DNA. The ease with which researchers could perform DNA sequencing meant that a lot of scientists got on board. Everybody was sequencing DNA and churning out reams of interesting results. The process, called polymerase chain reaction (PCR), would be the foundation for a rapid expansion in the identification and studying of genes, which would win Mullis the 1993 Nobel Prize in Chemistry.

Today we sequence genes with much more sophisticated equipment that does it rapidly. One of the significant contributions that this kind of research has made is in the field of zoology, which was transformed by being able to tell what's related to what, like the trick of telling the difference between the French restaurant and the Chinese restaurant. By looking at the ingredients one could find the complete tree of family relationships, making it possible to get a lot of hard data, and a huge amount of good science suddenly became possible. Of course, people immediately looked at what medical applications this technology—and the information it created—could have.

But hard data like that derived by DNA sequencing could only go so far to explain certain things about us and our potential for illness. Although in some dramatic medical examples a disease is caused by a missing key ingredient, like the case of the French restaurant with no butter, most diseases aren't nearly as straightforward. Cystic fibrosis is a classic case where the problem resides in a single gene coding for a single protein. But if you really want to know what's going on in most diseases, you have to taste what's coming out of the kitchen. That's proteomics. Proteins are what genes make. They are the end product of the process. Some diseases involve a single gene that results in deadly proteins. Huntington's disease, a genetic disorder that killed legendary singer and songwriter Woody Guthrie, is another example of an illness stemming from a single gene's malfunction, which produces the particular proteins that give rise to the illness.

Now, I have to extend this restaurant analogy a bit because the proteins are not just the food. As noted above, they are the process. They are the words of the conversation that goes on in the kitchen. The human body has some amazing stuff in it, but what's even more interesting is the process that builds it, maintains it, and modifies it. That process comes out of an ongoing conversation that's happening within cells and between cells in all the parts of the body. What are these cells all saying to each other? Proteomics is about understanding these conversations, for each word in the body's massive conversation is a protein. Defined another way, proteomics is spying on the dynamic conversation going on within the body at any given moment.

Building Blocks to Life and Health

You may already have heard that proteins, and specifically their chemical units called amino acids, are the "building blocks to life." This is apt: proteins are essential parts of organisms and participate in virtually every process within cells. Many proteins are enzymes that catalyze biochemical reactions and are vital to metabolism. Proteins also have structural or mechanical functions, such as actin and myosin in muscle and the proteins in the cytoskeleton, which form a system of scaffolding that maintains cell shape. Other proteins are important in cell signaling, immune responses, cell adhesion, and the cell cycle. Because of the diverse roles that these organic compounds fulfill in the body, proteins are a core ingredient to life and health. The sequence of amino acids in a protein is defined by the sequence of a gene, which is of course encoded in the DNA. As with sequencing DNA, sequencing a protein is easy to do nowadays, but figuring out what that protein actually does in the body as a result— and how it affects other aspects of the body's system—is the harder part to decode.

Proteins are also necessary in our diets, since we, along with many other animals, cannot synthesize all the amino acids we need and must obtain essential amino acids from food. When we eat food, our bodies go to work breaking down proteins into their amino acids, which then get absorbed and transported by the blood to cells for use. It's true that we are what we eat. If we performed a complete chemical analysis of our bodies, the report would list materials similar to those in foods: water, fat molecules, carbohydrates, protein complexes, and vitamins and minerals that help us to metabolize food and generate the energy we need to live. Think of the body as a self-maintaining factory; it is constantly regenerating itself down to every cell. Each month we renew our skin, every six weeks we have a new liver, and every three months we have new bones.

What makes proteomics so magnificently powerful is that the body is perfectly plumbed for analyzing proteins methodically. Blood circulates through each of us, and the proteins found therein reflect everything going on in a global sense. So, if your toe is infected and you draw blood from your arm, the inflammation proteins from the toe would be visible there. Your overall well-being can theoretically be measured at any given time from any given location in your blood by an examination of your proteins. The challenge, however, is being able to decipher the true meaning of all proteins, and how they work in conjunction with each other to either drive your body toward or away from health. That's where a field such as proteomics comes into play. Though it might seem easy for us to solve complicated health questions and problems through studying proteins, the body's mysteries remain shrouded for many reasons.

The Potential Power of Proteomics

In the medical field, we've known for a long time that it would be fantastic to be able to "listen" to all the proteins our bodies create. We just haven't been able to do this well. This endeavor is technically much, much more difficult than genomics. One reason is that the dynamic range of proteins in each of us in tremendous; there's ten to twelve orders of magnitude in difference between the most commonly found proteins in the body and the rare proteins. What you also have to keep in mind is that the technology used to study proteins looks at differences between protein fragments at the resolution level of an individual neutron, which is imperceptibly small. It's a mighty challenge to study such intricate and delicately small pieces of information without producing errors that skew results.

Unlike the case with genomics, we can't just add a few ingredients together to generate an easy readout of your proteins. To the contrary, the collecting and organizing of these massive molecules is essentially an analog—not a digital—process, just as I mentioned earlier that the human body is an analog object, not a digital one. It matters how much of each protein there is, and among hundreds of thousands of protein variants active in a system, the amounts of specific proteins present at any given instant can differ by many orders of magnitude.

Scientists have tried for years to measure all the proteins in a laboratory, but it was just too hard. The measurements were noisy and unrepeatable. A measurement would not give the same result a second time, which made producing any kind of reliable, provable result impossible. This gave proteomics a bad name—people started to give up trying to study more than a few proteins at a time, dismissing it as a useless endeavor. But I believed that eventually the technology would be able to meet the challenge, and that proteomics could offer great possibility to the world of medicine, which was desperately seeking innovation. My field of cancer research, in particular, ached for fresh insights.

In attempting to meet this challenge, one of the hurdles to confront is the sensitivity of the process to study the body's proteins. You can't just walk into the lab at 9:00 a.m., conduct an experiment with a sample of blood that any fifth-grader can follow, then have a machine spit out a report card of the analysis in a couple of hours. That's more like DNA sequencing these days. Unfortunately, analyzing the proteins in blood entails hundreds of steps, and any misstep along the way will affect your results. So, if you're doing this with graduate students in a bio lab, and one of them goes and changes the radio station at one step and leaves the sample fifteen seconds longer in a chemical, you get a completely different result. This is unacceptable in science. If you cannot get repeatable results, you might as well hang up your hat and call it a day. Repeatable results are what allow us to draw reliable conclusions.

Hence Al Gore's insistence that I allow Danny Hillis to help me solve my problem. At its core, ours was an engineering problem, and this meant that it was probably not going to be solved by biologists such as me. My experiment needed some better physics. It needed some tightly controlled engineering, something that looked more like a semiconductor line than a lab bench, with many steps that had to be refined and controlled to get a repeatable result. Besides, even if we could measure hundreds of thousands of protein levels, making any sense of them also created a huge mathematical problem—a computing problem. Each picture of the proteins in an individual patient yields an image of almost forty gigabytes. I would need Hillis for more than just the initial stages, and though

I won't bore you with the details of how much engineering has been involved, suffice it to say that it has called on all of our expertise. The solution has involved robotics; parallel computing, which is a form of computation in which many calculations are carried out simultaneously ("in parallel"); and changing the mass spectrometers that weigh proteins.

The mechanics of mass spectrometry is pretty simple. To measure the characteristics of individual molecules, a mass spectrometer converts them to ions, which are charged particles, so that they can be moved about and manipulated by external electrical and magnetic fields. A sample is ionized, the ions are sorted and separated according to their mass and charge, then these separated ions are measured, the results of which can be displayed on a chart. With proteins, which tend to be large molecules, the mass spectrometers first smash them into fragments of amino acid chains, which are then sorted by mass. We compare the results of a given sample to databases of known or predicted protein fingerprints to identify the original, parent protein. That's the short version of the story, because a lot more engineering goes on to arrive at digital pictures of human proteins. The science of this technology is straightforward, but the perfect execution of all this technology in concert, especially when dealing with human samples that can quickly change, is anything but!

By 2009, we had our assembly line set up after about six years of painstaking work. It performs these hundreds of steps automatically, and for the first time we can obtain results that are accurate and repeatable. We can take a drop of blood and identify more than a hundred thousand features of that blood—features that appear to be the same from person to person.

Let's actually look at a drop of blood that has gone through a superconducting magnet, giving us enough detail to begin to see all of the proteins in the body. We can start to see that system—the much bigger picture as a whole.

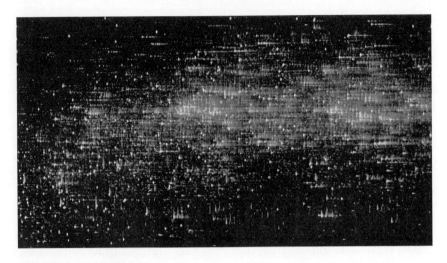

Source: Applied Proteomics.

This may look like a constellation of stars, but it's actually a high-resolution picture of the human proteome. This represents the equivalent of a 70,000-megapixel camera shot of a drop of blood. In other words, we're looking at a "picture" of the proteins swirling around this person's blood, which includes measurements at the atomic level of such complexity that it devours about forty gigabytes of storage space to hold all of the sample data (and this picture represents only about one twenty-fourth of the total data from the sample). The colors (not shown here) are used to indicate the abundance of a protein at a given position in the three-dimensional space, with the most abundant proteins appearing to be "closer" in the starry field. We don't know necessarily what all of these features (i.e., the dots and flecks) are, but we can identify many thousands of them as known proteins, and we now have genes associated with them. Often that means we know something about their function, such as a protein that aids in the metabolism of caffeine, or where the proteins are created in the body (e.g., the stomach), and so on. A good analogy to use in understanding the power of this technology is to think of Google Earth on steroids. We can zoom in on a single dot, identify that dot as a protein found in cold-water fish, and infer that the person could have eaten salmon or halibut for lunch. Of course, we would want to make more useful and insightful conclusions, such as whether a certain protein points to something abnormal going on in the body, or a strange pattern of proteins that forecasts disease. And that's exactly what this technology promises to achieve as our understanding of proteins—and our library of knowledge in the database—grows bigger.

Imagine what we can now do with this information. We can see differences between one person and another, not just the difference in the parts list, but also the difference in what is actually happening *inside* them. As I've been reiterating, DNA is static, but proteins are dynamic. They change in your body every minute depending on what's going on internally. At my laboratories at the Center for Applied Molecular Medicine at USC and Applied Proteomics, the company I cofounded with Danny Hillis, this is the kind of work we're doing—trying to find the key to understanding all of our body's proteins and how they work together to create the language our bodies speak, which ultimately translates the dialogue of our health.

The goal is to discover tests for certain illnesses based on proteins. The first commercial applications of proteomics will be diagnostics, and what's called theragnostics, which looks at markers that predict outcome to therapies. So an oncologist such as me could have a proteomic test for cancer, which looks for certain blood markers—proteins in the blood that indicate something unusual or abnormal going on—to identify changes in the state of the body that we can then address, or to be able to predict the response to a drug or surgery in a patient. This would take the place of invasive techniques used today such as biopsies. Proteomics could clue doctors into better ways of treating and whether invasive steps need to be taken at all.

Proteomic-based tests aren't as new as you might think. We have used them for decades, but in the past they have been employed to look at individual proteins, nothing more. One of the first proteomic tests developed was to study the level of human chorionic gonadotropin (HCG), a hormone secreted by a pregnant woman soon after fertilization. In the early part of the twentieth century, pregnancy testing involved injecting a woman's urine into the ear vein of a female rabbit. Then, a lab tech would examine the ovaries of that rabbit several days later. If the woman's urine contained the hormone HCG, then the rabbit ovaries would change in response to the hormone and indicate a positive pregnancy. The "rabbit test" became a widely used bioassay (animal-based test) to test for pregnancy. Then, at the end of 1977, Warner Chilcott marketed the first over-the-counter home pregnancy test to consumers called the e.p.t. (Early Pregnancy Test) for about $10, and thousands of rabbits rejoiced.

But let's think about other applications for this kind of analysis of proteins: Let's say I could find a pattern of proteins expressed in your blood that said whether your colon was growing polyps. That would be much better than having a colonoscopy to see if polyps, the abnormal growths of tissue that can become cancerous, are present. People are currently told to get a colonoscopy every five or ten years after a certain age, but one in a thousand people will experience serious damage from the procedure itself, not to mention plenty of trepidation beforehand. Unfortunately, at this point we don't have a better way of telling if your colon is in a precancerous stage. If you could find that out through an annual blood test, however, wouldn't that be much better and easier to endure? You would only undergo a colonoscopy if you had an actual polyp that needed to be removed. This is just one example of the possibilities that proteomics can afford us. Health care costs would inevitably come down, and the risk of secondary harm from invasive techniques would also diminish, if not totally vanish.

Doctors today are limited in lots of ways by current technology.

Often a doctor can only determine whether a lump is cancerous via a biopsy. Ovarian cancer, for example, is hard to diagnose early. Imagine a series of minimally invasive technologies that can aid in arriving at proper diagnosis early and can inform effective treatment. In the case of ovarian cancer, there'd be a simple blood test that a woman can have every year during her annual Pap that looks for certain proteins in the blood that indicate the early stages of ovarian cancer. That's the promise of a field such as proteomics, which will likely join a broad platform of emerging technologies designed to revolutionize medicine.

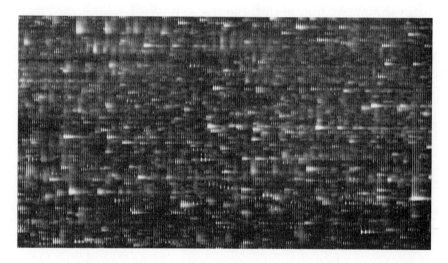

Proteomic analysis of two individuals layered on top of each other. If you were to see this in color, one person's set would be red and the other green. When they match exactly they are yellow. Source: Applied Proteomics.

Complex Systems Medicine

As with genomics, a great deal of decoding still needs to be done until we're at a point where you can get your proteins profiled and draw useful conclusions. We don't know what all of these features that we've found in blood mean or how they relate to one another. It may be that, like a genetic test, some single feature will actually tell us something important. But probably much more of the information lies in the patterns and combinations that we find. It's almost as if we're in the Gregor Mendel and Charles Darwin phase, toiling with our experiments and taking as many notes as we can to solve the ultimate puzzle of understanding the human body and the innumerable ways in which it conducts business for health or sickness. One of the major differences between how we're working today and how Darwin and Mendel operated from their respective corners of the world more than a hundred years ago, is that we're not working in a vacuum. As I write this, the research is being performed by a consortium of people in such places as Stanford, Caltech, the Santa Fe Institute, the University of Washington, Arizona State University, Translational Genomics Institute in Phoenix, Cold Spring Harbor Laboratory in New York, Applied Proteomics, and at my teams' labs at USC.

Ten or twenty years from now, a droplet of blood may be all that your doctor needs to catch a fomenting illness, even cancer, in its earliest stages. That droplet might also reveal which genetic diseases you are at risk of developing later in life and which medicines, tailored to your genetic makeup and personal physiology, are right for you. We can start to develop blood products and start to intervene earlier.

Without a question, sometime in the future our individual genome sequences, or at least sections of them, will be part of our medical files, and routine blood tests will involve thousands of measurements to test for various diseases and genetic predispositions to other conditions. Medicine will shift from being heavily trafficked on the treatment side to the prevention side, rooted in science-based predictions. What will make this all possible is the universal embrace of complex systems medicine, which blends biology, computing, engineering, and a layer of rationale from the physics world to try to understand the behavior of a "whole" (as in the whole human body) in terms of the interactions among its parts—its genes, its proteins, and any other molecules that play a defining role.

Throughout history, the field of engineering evolved to levels at which it can control complex systems without necessarily understanding them. In my field of medicine, unfortunately, we've taken another approach. As you know by now, I believe that we've spent far too long focusing on understanding but not controlling. I yearn to see the day when we can operate more like how they do at high-tech computer companies. At Sun Microsystems, for example, which was acquired by Oracle in 2009, engineers could predict where a system was going to fail before it happened and swap out the faulty component before it brought the whole system down. Imagine if we had that kind of capability in medicine. You'd first have to know where to look—where vulnerable areas are and how to check for potential flaws or future failures—and then know how to optimize conditions to prevent any malfunction. You could also, in essence, swap out the "components" that aren't functioning properly or that need a tune-up through drug therapies or modifications in your lifestyle that target those allegorical components. So rather than treating illness or breakdowns in the system after the fact, you're effectively preventing failures from happening.

At the heart of complex systems medicine is this idea that you want to identify the elements of a system and measure their interactions and relationships as you "perturb" the system. Disease, after all, is a "perturbation" of the system by either genetic or environmental changes, or both. Once we have mapped out the full network of genes or proteins that interact in a certain type of tissue, we can tweak pieces of the network in different samples and compare the results. For example, we can test out what blood-pressure medication or a daily baby aspirin is doing to the system overall, and in areas where we wouldn't suspect such drugs are having an impact. Ultimately, these sorts of experiments may turn up molecular changes involved in cancer, inflammation, or any number of other conditions. In many cases, these changes may include proteins that cells secrete into the bloodstream, which is where the idea of a blood test for diseases including cancer comes in.

Before long, not only will drug companies be developing personalized therapies, but doctors will be able to change how they dispense drugs and determine who gets what treatment. For example, let's say that we try out a drug on cancer patients, and we find out that only 20 percent of them respond to the drug. It's a useless drug if it doesn't help most people, and it might even make some people very sick. Wouldn't it be nice if we knew about a pattern of proteins or other molecules in the blood that told us which 20 percent responded to the drug? After all, it's a miracle drug for those 20 percent. If genetics alone could tell you who would respond to which drugs, then we wouldn't need the information from proteins and other molecules. But this part of medicine doesn't depend on those parts lists. By and large, that kind of information doesn't just depend on the ingredients list; it depends on what is happening in the kitchen.

The valuable information is much more likely to be in the proteins. We can start to say, "If we see pattern X in the proteins, it means that you've got problem Y, and drug Z would help." All of a sudden we've got hundreds of thousands of indicators to tell us what's actually going on in the body—and whether it's being driven toward or away from health. We can, for the first time, really examine, measure, and understand our system. Which can mean all the difference when it comes to the future of medicine as well as your future well-being.

Certainly, some other kinds of molecules are important, too. It's not just proteins. We know, for example, that glucose is important. Glucose is a sugar molecule that drives cellular metabolism; it's our chief source of energy. But proteins regulate the production and breakdown of other molecules such as glucose, so if we have an understanding of all the proteins' state, then we can infer what's going on with those other molecules. Granted, the body's overall state doesn't solely rely on its proteins, but most of the information seems to be there. I believe that if we can comprehend the language created by proteins, we can accomplish a lot.

For someone such as me, this is an exciting era in medicine because, with the help of advanced technology and the application of engineering principles and systems thinking, for the first time we're able to look at the variables of this complex process—the dynamic variables, which is what life is.

The Future You: Taking Treatment Personally

Whatever the treatment of cancer or autoimmune disease, neuro-degenerative disease or other system diseases, will be like in the future, it will likely be individually created for you. The diagnosis won't necessarily dictate your treatment. Instead, a combination of imaging techniques and blood work will examine your proteins plus any other important details. From that, your doctors will be able to build a model of your "state"— a portrait of the state of your health and your body's dynamics. They will also be able to monitor your systemic state's progress. This will include your genes, your metabolites—which are molecules formed in your body as part of your metabolism—and the proteins that communicate between your cells. A dynamic time model will note what the cells are saying to each other, what molecules are being produced at a faster or slower rate, and so on. Then, from this model your doctors will actually simulate your specific body under lots of different treatment scenarios; they'll simulate for your cancering and learn how you can tweak your body back into a healthy state. The treatment will be very specific. Your doctor may treat you in a very different way than he's ever treated any other human before, but the model will say that, for you, that's the proper treatment.

This kind of personalized medicine isn't as far off into the future as you might think. It's already gaining momentum in the field of psychiatry, which is historically rife with exhausting episodes of blind trial and error. The genetics of mental illness are still a maddeningly complex mystery, but luckily progress is being made by taking an approach like the one I've been advocating since the beginning of this book. Rather than trying to understand depression, doctors are successfully controlling it through targeted drug therapies.

People respond differently to drugs, as is the case with antidepressants, and doctors must search to find the ideal type and dose for each individual patient. When psychiatrists set out to prescribe an antidepressant, they have no clinically proven way of knowing which one to choose. Any given antidepressant tends to help only about a third of patients; the other two-thirds end up doing the prescription shuffle, trying one drug, then another, then a third or fourth in hopes of finally hitting on a treatment that works.

Several new tests are being used that identify variants in multiple genes and tell doctors which antidepressant to pick based on their results, which is part of a first wave of long-awaited pharmacogenomic progress—pharmacogenomics, you'll recall, is the subfield of personalized medicine that focuses on how people with different DNA variants respond to drugs. The DNA tests I referred to previously perform pharmacogenomic tests to a variety of therapeutics, such as blood thinners, cancer drugs, and antibiotics, but the newer, specialized tests for psychiatric disorders are also being used to manage patients today. These tests have recently become standard of care or similar at the Mayo Clinic and Cincinnati Children's Hospital Medical Center, the two institutions where one of the tests was developed. At the Mayo, doctors have for three decades been laying the basic-research groundwork for how this test could be used in both adults and children. And it's not just about treating depression. A list of drugs pages long are metabolized by the same proteins used to process antidepressants. If you have your DNA screened, you can know how well your body responds to these drugs and whether, for example, you should have a higher-than-average dose of blood thinner to start a particular therapy based on how your body metabolizes the drug. In other words, your genetic report will also include valuable information about how to customize drugs to your metabolism. Hopefully, you'll never need the information on the drugs listed in these tests, but the likelihood is we'll all have medical issues at some point, and the dosing of these drugs can be calculated much more individually if your physician has the profile of your metabolism genes.

In 2010, *Newsweek* published an article that explained this advancement in very practical terms. Rightfully so, it stated that "although [we] know fairly little about the genetics of mental illness, [we] know much more about genes that influence the way the body processes drugs." The Mayo and Cincinnati researchers developed a particular expertise around a group of enzymes referred to as the "cytochrome P450 superfamily," or CYP450 for short, which help the liver metabolize many chemicals. If you have certain variants in the genes that make proteins in the CYP450 group, your body may process a drug faster or, conversely, slower than other people. Either the drug's effects wear off quickly or last a long time.

The genetic tests on the market can then utilize that knowledge. One, called the GeneSightRx, for example, tests for five genes; three of its five genes code for proteins involved in the CYP450 pathway. The other two code for variants in the brain's serotonin receptors and transporters, respectively. So far, twelve thousand patients at Mayo and Cincinnati Children's have been assessed with GeneSightRx and have had their drugs tailored to their individual metabolisms.

In theory, your family doctor or psychiatrist could do all this without GeneSightRx, by employing a test such as one done by Navigenics. The problem, as duly noted in *Newsweek*, is that your doctor would then have to comb through the scientific literature looking for references to how your particular variants affect the metabolism of different drugs, then evaluate several antidepressants by searching the literature some more and choose one for you accordingly. By the time you read this, the test will likely have expanded to include more genes to the profile it can provide. As we decode more and more genes and add them to the test, it will become a more reliable guide for picking medications. My personal test results done with my company are shown below with the drugs being tested today, indicating both the effectiveness of a select group of drugs as well as the side effects of other drugs.

(This is the actual report I received; again, the footnotes are speaking to me.)

Medication Side Effects

Drug[1]	Side effect[2]	Your risk[3]
Carbamazepine (Carbatrol®)	Life-threatening dermatological syndromes that include fever, rash, and peeling skin.	low risk
Fluorouracil (Efudex®)	Severe, potentially fatal toxicity	low risk
Irinotecan (Camptosar®)	Severe reactions, including suppression of the immune system	low risk
Simvastatin (Vytorin®, Zocor®)	Muscle pain and damage	low risk
Succinylcholine (Anectine®)	Prolonged, potentially dangerous paralysis of the breathing muscles	low risk
Thiopurines (Azasan®)	Severe bone marrow complications	low risk

[1]**Drug:** We analyzed your genetic code to determine how effective this medication is for you.
[2]**Side effect:** Severe side effects associated with this medication.
[3]**Your risk:** Your risk of side effects, based on the markers we found in your generic code.

Medication Effectiveness

Drug[1]	Information[2]	How effective for you[3]
Beta blockers (Coreg®, many others)	Used to treat and prevent cardiovascular disease	typical effectiveness
Clopidogrel (Plavix®)	Used to prevent blood clots and conditions linked to them, such as heart attack and stroke	decreased effectiveness
Statins (Pravachol®, Zocor®, many others)	Used to treat high cholesterol and help prevent heart disease	decreased cholesterol lowering, but some cardiac effectiveness
Warfarin (Coumadin®)	Used to treat and prevent blood clots and heart-related conditions, such as atrial fibrillation and heart attack	standard dose

[1]**Drug:** We analyzed your genetic code to determine how effective this medication is for you.
[2]**Information:** Medical conditions for which this drug is commonly used.
[3]**How effective for you:** How effective this medication is for you, based on the markers we found in your genetic code.
Source: Navigenics.

Being able to continuously measure and adjust the balance of drugs in a living system will transform the pharmaceutical industry, making it into a much more science-based endeavor than one of trial and error. It would be a shame if you were taking the correct drug, but the dose was too low for your inherited metabolism and you didn't benefit from the drug. In addition, advances that a field such as proteomics can offer will help us to gain control of diseases that take a long time to develop. Easing depression is unlike other afflictions that can take much longer to fulminate, evolve, and treat. Right now, for example, we can't tell what's happening in a body until an underlying, manifesting disease progresses to the point that it causes a noticeable symptom. If you have an ailment that takes a long time to play out, such as Alzheimer's disease, or amyotrophic lateral sclerosis (ALS, better known as Lou Gehrig's disease), we don't know if your drug is doing any good for years and years. We also don't know if the dosage is too high. But if you could actually look at the proteins and notice this bad problem of communication between the cells, which is causing plaque formation in the brain in the case of Alzheimer's disease, then you might be able to see the response to the drug immediately, even though the symptoms aren't changing yet. The symptoms may take years to change or even surface, but we can see the drug is effective in you immediately . . . or that it's not, so we can move on to trying the next drug.

Of course this type of innovation will also find its way into the world of nutrition. Once again, when you consider traditional Chinese or ayurvedic medicine, or any approach to eating that looks at how the body should be fed to maintain a balance and to restore any forces working against it, there's never been a true model behind such a method. Now, with the twin powers of genomics and proteomics, we can finally begin to inject some science into the art of good nutrition. If you had a much better, evidence-based model, then you could probably rationally understand what foods you should be eating to bring your body back into balance. Whether that means you'll choose to eat those foods is another story, but at least you'll have a better idea of what you personally can do. And then it's really up to you.

Health Rule

Know as much about yourself as possible through the use of technology, including how you metabolize drugs. Technology has allowed us to live long enough to develop age-related disease. It also will allow us to prevent, treat, and manage age-related disease so we can live robustly for as long as possible.

PART II

The Elements of Healthy Style

The only way to keep your health is to eat what you don't want, drink what you don't like, and do what you'd rather not.

—*Mark Twain*

In 1918, William Strunk Jr. wrote *The Elements of Style* to help guide his students in their writings at Cornell University, where he was a professor of English. It was privately published the following year, but didn't become a perennial bestseller until writer E. B. White, who had studied under Strunk, revised and expanded the book for a 1959 edition. Asserting that one must first know the rules to break them, this now classic reference, widely known as simply "Strunk and White," is considered by many to be a must-have for conscientious writers. With nuances of humor, toughness, irreverence, and a no-holds-barred approach to good grammar all wrapped into a quick read, the book offers a blend of rules to write by, as well as advice for developing one's own writing style.

Where am I going with this? Much in the way Strunk and White so marvelously conveyed the principles of English style while attacking common violations and putting to bed myths related to the use of language, my hope in this next part is to similarly attack certain mythologies that perpetually swirl in health and wellness circles, and to help you develop and live by your own healthy style. By "style," I mean the things you can do to use all the knowledge we currently have in medicine to design a custom plan for your unique body. By establishing your baseline, you've already gotten a head start to defining your personal metrics. Now, with the information you gain in the upcoming sections, you'll be able to further fine-tune your personal metrics as you see fit. Your goal is to continually shift the balance to a healthy state of being.

You cannot prevent every ailment and disease, but when you start to employ tactical strategies to improving your health in the ways that I'll be describing, you can change your state of health for the better. You can slowly extricate yourself from the superstitions and ignorance that could be interfering with your achievement of total health. An ounce of prevention is worth more than a million pounds of cure.

Over the years, the idea of what is healthy has dramatically changed; advertisements in the 1950s used to proclaim the benefits of doctor-approved cigarette brands or of products such as margarine. While I believe in direct-to-consumer advertising, I also think that we have to be careful. As they did in the past, and still do to this day, drug companies and marketers and hawkers of all things "good for you" tend to get it all wrong, and they tend to do this in the name of profit, rather than an interest in what is actually good for us. It goes back to the notion of a metric. When it comes to promoting health, pharmaceutical companies and doctors typically show only one metric. Are these smart metrics upon which to base our decisions? Probably not.

What is your metric? You will be able to answer that ultimate question as I further show you how to be your own advocate for personal health. As I hope I've proved thus far, health is dynamic. It's so dynamic as to be a verb, not a noun. So let's find out what you can do to engage in health and prevent as many ill outcomes as possible. We'll first turn to some of our most trusted companions in the quest for health: vitamins. And we'll start with the most popular one of late, vitamin D, which you'll note I didn't list on the tests to get in creating your baseline.

6

Proceed with Caution

Studies, Claims, and Scare Tactics

I magine a treatment that builds bones, strengthens the immune system, averts depression and fibromyalgia, clears up psoriasis, and lowers the risk of illnesses such as diabetes, heart and kidney disease, high blood pressure, and even cancer. Oh, and it also helps you to sleep better at night and dodge insomnia. This might sound too good to be true, but some research suggests that such a miracle cure already exists. It's vitamin D, a nutrient that the body makes from sunlight and that is also found in wild fish and fortified foods such as milk and even margarine.

When I googled the term *vitamin D* in the summer of 2011, the search engine turned up 24.4 million results, many of which linked to studies of this vitamin. Vitamin D was discovered nearly a century ago, but it has become a media darling in recent years. I hardly need to point out that health-related headlines of any kind tend to sprawl and become seemingly more important. And when they speak to counterintuitive wisdom or somehow show a serious flaw in our quest for health, these announcements spread rapidly and demand attention. Vitamin D's rise to fame illustrates a classic case of how we can fall prey to hype that's fairly one-sided, and lacking substantial data. I'm going to use the case of vitamin D to show how easy it is to buy into extravagant claims, but the same can be said for a lot of health claims. My intention is to motivate you to be skeptical of studies and question all assertions related to health. I've made vitamin D the fall guy here because its story is so rich in important biological themes and symbolic of how many of us accept incoming information like dogma. It affords me the opportunity to demonstrate just how naive and narrow-minded we can be with regard to bold promises in health circles.

From Headlines to Health Alerts

Let's look at a few examples of headlines about vitamin D that have circulated lately:

Lack of Vitamin D in Patients with Leukemia "Ups Death Risk"

Vitamin D Proven Far Better Than Vaccines at Preventing Influenza Infections

Low Vitamin D Levels Linked to Parkinson's Disease

Vitamin D Halts Growth of Breast Cancer Tumors

Vitamin D Prevents Breast Cancer

Vitamin D Prevents Heart Disease

Vitamin D Really Does Prevent Cancer, Autoimmune Diseases

Vitamin D Protects Against Strokes

Sixty Million Years of Evolution Says Vitamin D May Save Your Life from Swine Flu

Low Vitamin D Levels Linked to Poor Blood Sugar Control in Type 2 Diabetes

Breast Cancer Virtually "Eradicated" with Higher Levels of
   Vitamin D
Vitamin D Promotes Weight Loss
Vitamin D Deficiency May Be to Blame for Chronic Hives

And my personal favorite: *New Research Shows Vitamin D Slashes Risk of Cancers by 77 Percent; Cancer Industry Refuses to Support Cancer Prevention*

If the words *prevent, protects, proven, save your life, eradicated,* and *weight loss* grabbed your attention, you're not alone. Sales of vitamin D supplements in the United States have soared in recent years, and clinical laboratory testing for 25-hydroxyvitamin D—the specific vitamin D metabolite in the body used as an indicator of one's vitamin D status—continues to be the fastest-growing test on the medical-laboratory menu in the United States and other developed nations worldwide. The steady increase in physician and patient demand for vitamin D tests has kept most pathology laboratories scrambling to maintain turnaround times and quality. In some parts of Canada, labs have shut down testing because the demand is too high for the budgets allowed by the country's public health-care system.

What fuels sustained demand for vitamin D testing are two powerful trends. First is news that a significant number of individuals have insufficient levels of vitamin D (another headline of late: *Epidemic of Vitamin D Deficiency Sweeping the World*). With surprising regularity, major media outlets in the United States publish or broadcast stories featuring interviews with physicians and health experts who tell the American public that a high number of people suffer from a vitamin D deficiency. Just those words alone—*deficient* and *insufficient*—are enough to inspire any well-intentioned individual to seek a remedy. In my own practice, virtually all the patients I see exhibit some level of vitamin D deficiency. Among the US population, according to the most recently analyzed National

Health and Nutrition Examination Survey data, only 23 percent of US adolescents and adults had serum vitamin D levels of 30 nanograms per milliliter (ng/mL) or more, which is the level considered "adequate" or "normal." Nearly all non-Hispanic blacks (97%) and most Mexican-Americans (90%) are characterized as vitamin D "insufficient" (level less than 30 ng/mL).

The second trend has been the persistent headlines that scream how beneficial adequate levels of vitamin D can be for human health. From lowering your risk for cancer to helping you stave off infections and colds, vitamin D practically has its own PR campaign today courtesy of this relentless press coverage and volume of published clinical studies in academia that connect low vitamin D levels with a growing number of disease and health conditions. In early 2010, for example, the *British Medical Journal* published the results of a case control study conducted by the European Prospective Investigation into Cancer and Nutrition (EPIC) that found that people whose vitamin D levels were in the top fifth had a 40 percent lower risk for colorectal cancer than those in the bottom fifth. Within a month, another study published in *Arthritis & Rheumatism* determined that older men with insufficient vitamin D levels had twice the likelihood of showing signs of hip osteoarthritis on an X-ray than those with normal levels.

So if you're like many who've been caught up in this recent health-alert blitzkrieg, you've either gotten your vitamin D levels checked and begun a daily supplement regimen, or you've gone ahead and purchased a bottle of vitamin D with the thought that it won't hurt—and just might help. I don't fault you for doing this. What person is going to disagree with all of this well-documented literature and the phalanx of advanced-degreed scientists from prestigious institutions who are churning out scores of data and associations between low vitamin D levels and illness?

Therein resides one of the problems: we're talking about *associations* and related verbiage that can confuse and mislead the lay public. What's more, amid the flurry of articles lionizing vitamin D, it's easy to miss some of the other headlines pitching another side to the story. Three cases in point:

Vitamin D Fails Osteoarthritis Test: In a two-year study, vitamin D supplements failed to reduce pain or slow the progression of joint damage in people with osteoarthritis of the knee.

Annual Vitamin D Dose Linked to Increased Fall, Fracture Risk in Older Women: According to the results of a double-blind, placebo-controlled trial reported in the May 12, 2010, issue of the *Journal of the American Medical Association*, older women living in the same community who received annual oral high-dose vitamin D had an *increased* risk for falls and fractures. Double-blind, placebo-controlled studies are highly valued; they are the gold standard for clinical studies because neither the participants nor the researchers know who received the real thing or the placebo, an inactive pill that looked like the vitamin, until the experiment is complete. This guards against bias.

Serum Vitamin D Concentration and Prostate Cancer Risk: In 2008, the *Journal of the National Cancer Institute* published an analysis of the relationship between prostate cancer risk and serum 25-hydroxyvitamin D level in aging men. The results of this study prompted the researchers to conclude that vitamin D does not reduce the risk of prostate cancer, and furthermore that higher circulating levels of 25-hydroxyvitamin D may be associated with an *increased* risk of more aggressive forms of prostate cancer.

Reading Between the Lines to Find Another Side to the Story

How can this be? Why the conflicting reports? Vitamin D, is, after all, supposed to support bone health and thus protect against falls and fractures. What explains the discrepancy? It turns out, as with most things in life, the case for vitamin D isn't a slam dunk and it's far from straightforward. One of the reasons is that while vitamin D may appear to be an anticancer miracle worker in the lab where you can control cell cultures much better, and where it's been shown to halt tumor growth, this effect doesn't replicate itself in live people. When you read a headline that states "Vitamin D Halts Growth of Breast Cancer Tumors," you have to ask a critical question: how was this proven? This was an actual headline published at NaturalNews.com, and among the proof provided was that "vitamin D cream can be rubbed directly on tumors to make them vanish." If vitamin D cream were a cure for some forms of cancer, don't you think we'd all know about this by now? The same goes for any other concoction of vitamin D; if it were an antidote to cancer, it would have been declared the most important discovery of our generation. The body and its vitamin D system are a lot more complicated than that. Keep in mind that what can be proven in a cell culture or petri dish doesn't always translate to live human subjects.

Numerous studies have shown no benefit for vitamin D in cancer patients, and one study in particular came to a screeching end in 2007 when giving high doses of calcitriol (a potent form of vitamin D) to patients with advanced prostate cancer caused an "imbalance of deaths" between those given the drug and the placebo group. The people who received the regimen with vitamin D oddly outpaced the placebo group in their death count. Did the vitamin D somehow hasten the deaths of these individuals? Tumors, like any other organ in the body, contain vitamin D receptors, which are the molecules that allow vitamin D to attach to cells and have an effect. Some studies have shown that these receptors can signal the tumor to slow down its growth, but what about *accelerating* growth? If vitamin D can nourish a healthy cell to help its development, then isn't it reasonable to think it could do this for a cancerous cell? Whether a study points to the benefits or potential downside to vitamin D, I'm not suggesting that these studies are necessarily wrong or flawed, though some of them might be. What I do want to emphasize is that the confusion and conflicting information are worthy of speculation and further analysis. We just don't have all the clues yet to make any definitive answer on the matter, which can be said for many nutrients that are marketed as superstar health promoters.

True marked vitamin D deficiency manifests in bone conditions, the most famous of which—childhood rickets—became the rallying cry for science to find out why we need the sun for survival. When the industrial revolution moved families from farms to factories, pioneering doctors noticed that the serious bone deformities of childhood rickets were epidemic in polluted European cities but not in rural areas. At the time, they treated the disease by prescribing exposure to sunlight, but they were ignored by the medical community until X-rays proved the case in the 1920s. The US government then recommended limited sun for children, and dairies began fortifying products with vitamin D, hence the labels we see today on containers of orange juice and milk.

Rickets disappeared, and in the twentieth century scientists eventually discovered how vitamin D works in the body. First, your skin absorbs UVB sunlight, which then triggers a cascade of events that leads to vitamin D's being activated in the kidneys for use by the body's organs and tissues. In addition to being necessary for maintaining your body's calcium levels, which in turn affects the health of your skeleton, vitamin D is also thought to regulate about two thousand genes in different ways. It plays a role in cell growth and death, which explains its connection to cancer. It affects blood vessels, linking it to blood pressure and heart health. Its involvement with inflammation and the immune system brings an association with allergies and asthma, infections such as influenza and tuberculosis, and autoimmune disorders such as multiple sclerosis and type 1 diabetes. The higher the level of vitamin D in the system, the theory goes, the lower one's risk for these conditions.

But despite its role in many of the body's vital functions, we must be careful about making broad statements about vitamin D and its link ("associations") to various illnesses and disease. Despite thousands of studies, there's not a lot of strong research showing consistent benefits from vitamin D supplementation; and here, semantics again comes into play. "Studies" should mean large, controlled, double-blind, randomized trials that honor the scientific method. That doesn't always happen, especially with regard to vitamin D.

Performing a true study on vitamin D's potential benefit, which should theoretically result in reliable conclusions, is nearly impossible since vitamin D cannot be controlled in any given person. First, we have the stumbling block of dealing with a vitamin that can be obtained naturally from sunlight and certain foods such as wild salmon and fortified milk and cereals. Unlike a new drug that can be administered (i.e., controlled) in a specific manner to a group of participants, vitamin D cannot be allocated so easily to then determine benefits. If I give some vitamin D to one group of people but not the other one, and the other group is exposed to more sunlight or eats more foods rich in vitamin D, it becomes difficult, if not impossible, to compare the groups.

Let's take one of the more striking recent findings on vitamin D, which was presented by a team at the Intermountain Medical Center in Utah in 2009. Among the study's 27,686 patients at least fifty years old who had a vitamin D test in the last decade, heart failure was 90 percent more common in those with the lowest versus the highest levels; a previous heart attack was 81 percent more likely; a previous stroke was 51 percent more likely. So is there a connection? On the surface, the study would seem to make a strong case that vitamin D benefits people at risk for heart conditions.

An association, however, does not prove cause and effect. Another way of looking at this study is to say it's quite possible that a heart condition lowers vitamin D levels, directly or indirectly—by keeping people with health challenges indoors and out of the sun. Also, obesity throws another wrench into the problem because excess fat absorbs and holds on to vitamin D so that it cannot be properly used in the body. Hence, is low vitamin D in this study just a marker for those who were obese? It's the old chicken-and-egg conundrum. The same can be said for hundreds of other such studies that link the health (or lack thereof) of an individual to levels of vitamin D.

Another fact few researchers point out when they publish their studies on vitamin D is that virtually all of these studies have been observational. It may be that high doses of the nutrient don't make people healthier, but that healthy people do the sorts of things that raise vitamin D. According to JoAnn E. Manson, a Harvard professor who is chief of preventive medicine at Brigham and Women's Hospital in Boston, "People may have high vitamin D levels because they exercise a lot and are getting ultraviolet-light exposure from exercising outdoors. Or they may have high vitamin D because they are health conscious and take supplements. But they also have a healthy diet, don't smoke, and do a lot of the other things that keep you healthy."

Authors Steven Levitt and Stephen Dubner state clearly in their book *Freakonomics* what data can give us: elusive correlations. Data might seem to be incredibly rich and revealing, but that doesn't mean it's incredibly accurate, reliable, or that it tells the whole story. They write, "*Correlation is nothing more than a statistical term that indicates whether two variables move together. It tends to be cold outside when it snows; those two factors are positively correlated. Sunshine and rain, meanwhile, are negatively correlated. Easy enough—as long as there are only a couple of variables. But with a couple of hundred variables, things get harder.*" Indeed, things get so suspect as to be meaningless. And in the health world, we're dealing with an *infinite* number of variables. Low vitamin D may indicate that a person has a chronic condition such as obesity, but does it mean that the deficiency is causing obesity? We don't know.

Manson is currently leading a major study over the next several years that should shed more light on this confusing vitamin D topic. Her nationwide clinical trial is recruiting twenty thousand healthy older adults, including men sixty and older and women sixty-five and older, to study whether high doses of vitamin D and omega-3 fatty acids from fish-oil supplements will lower risk for heart disease and cancer. This has never before been done—there are currently no studies demonstrating that taking vitamin D lowers one's risk for illness, including cancer. Even the studies that point to higher incidences of cancer among those who live at higher latitudes (and who have lower levels of vitamin D) do not prove that vitamin D is to blame for these trends. Manson is questioning correlations like these, and she's not alone in her critical thinking.

The World Health Organization International Agency for Research on Cancer published a report in 2008 entitled "Vitamin D and Cancer." Its conclusions are compelling:

> Much of the data suggesting a link between vitamin D status and cancer have been derived from ecological studies that assessed the correlation between latitude and cancer mortality. However, causal inference from ecological studies is notoriously perilous as, among other things, these studies cannot adequately control for confounding by exposure to various cancer risk factors, which also vary with latitude (e.g., dietary habits or melatonin synthesis). Studies from the USA show a weak association between latitude and vitamin D status and that other factors such as outdoor activities and obesity are better predictive factors of vitamin D status. In Europe, the opposite has been found, with a south-to-north increase in serum 25-hydroxyvitamin D that parallels a similar gradient in the incidence of colorectal, breast, and prostate cancers.
>
> In people of the same age and skin complexion,

there is considerable interindividual variation in serum 25-hydroxyvitamin D even with similar levels of sun exposure. Overall, the evidence for breast cancer is limited, and there is no evidence for prostate cancer.

Two double-blind, placebo-controlled randomized trials (the Women's Health Initiative trial [WHI] in the USA and one smaller trial in the UK) showed that supplementation with vitamin D had no effect on colorectal or breast cancer incidence.

Clearly, we need to be careful about making unequivocal claims about the potential links between cancer incidence and highly variable things such as vitamin D. A medley of factors are likely at play, making it hard to reduce assertions down to truthful, black-and-white conclusions. Later in the book, for example, we'll explore the role that your microbiome, your intestinal bacteria, could be playing in your health equation, including your risk for cancer. Latitude doesn't affect just how much sun you get and your levels of vitamin D. This seemingly minor geographical circumstance can impact many aspects of your entire system, even when you exclude the influence of vitamin D.

Hopefully, studies like the one Manson is currently performing will increase in numbers around the world so we can arrive at more evidence-based conclusions. Manson is including fish-oil supplements in the study because they are another promising treatment that suffers from a dearth of good clinical-trial evidence. In addition, both vitamin D and fish oil are known to have an anti-inflammatory effect, though each works through a different pathway in the body, so there may be an added health benefit in combining them. Study participants will be divided into four groups. One will take both vitamin D and fish-oil pills. Two will take either a vitamin D or a fish-oil supplement and a placebo. The fourth will take two placebo pills. The study is expected to be complete around 2015.

Homeostatic Controls Always at Work Inside You

Benefits of vitamin D aside, the health of any person could be a factor of his or her lifestyle and other conditions that either raise or lower vitamin D levels. The body might lower vitamin D levels when it's faced with a particular condition. In the case of the Utah heart patients, for instance, did their condition lower their vitamin D or did their low vitamin D exacerbate their condition? We don't know, and this reiterates that the human body is a complex instrument for which we need better measurement systems. When we measure a single node in its intricate system, we are ignoring so many other nodes that likely have an impact in the body's overall functioning. Current methods of testing for vitamin D only look at one particular "junction" in the entire vitamin D system. How do I know that your body, for example, doesn't increase its vitamin D–making capacity somewhere else down the road?

The body is incredibly homeostatic. By that I mean that it has built-in mechanisms to preserve a stable, constant environment. The best example of this is our body's superior maintenance of temperature. As warm-blooded creatures, we like to be at roughly 98.6 degrees Fahrenheit. When we sway from this temperature, our biochemistry signals reactions to bring the temperature back to normal. While different body parts do have different temperatures and the time of day and certain conditions can affect your temperature, for the most part you will remain close to 98.6 degrees (barring any circumstance that can cause a dramatic spike or drop in temperature such as infection or a prolonged dip in icy waters).

Another prominent system in the body that abides by this rule of homeostasis is the regulation of your blood glucose, or sugar, in your bloodstream. All mammals regulate their blood sugar with the two hormones insulin and glucagon, and the human body maintains glucose levels constant most of the day—even after a twenty-four-hour fast. Anyone with diabetes understands that this system can be disrupted, requiring routine interventions to artificially maintain this homeostasis, which is the heart and soul of energy metabolism— turning food into fuel for the body's cellular processes. When the body can no longer regulate its blood-sugar metabolism, disease sets in and requires immediate attention. Diabetes is a breakdown in the body's system. In type 1, a person cannot produce insulin to move sugar out of the bloodstream and into cells for use; in type 2, an individual can produce insulin, but the cells become less responsive to the insulin so the movement of sugar out of the blood and into cells is less efficient. Both types of diabetes cause a serious interruption of physiological events meant to maintain a stable, steady, and well-fueled system.

Now, let's apply this knowledge of the body's desire for homeostasis to the vitamin D debate. Let's assume that, as with most of the other functions it performs, your body prefers to maintain stable levels of vitamin D. It can do so through your exposure to sunlight coupled with the vitamin D you eat. Due to the various shades of skin color, everyone has a different capacity to make vitamin D through the skin. Evolution made sure of this. People who are light skinned evolved in this fashion so they would be exposed to enough sunlight to maintain adequate levels of vitamin D, as they are often from regions with limited sun exposure. Conversely, those who live closer to the equator have ample opportunity to make vitamin D and thus evolved to have darker, more impenetrable skin. The more melanin in your skin, the darker you are and the harder it is to manufacture vitamin D. Melanin is the substance that gives your skin its color. This explains why dark-skinned people, such as African-Americans, are said to be at a much higher risk for vitamin D deficiency than their fair-skinned counterparts.

The recent vitamin D discussion, however, highlights that at this point in history mankind is geographically spread out and, in many cases, not living where evolution prepared us to thrive. But are displaced darkly complected people living in higher latitudes really suffering from dangerous vitamin D deficiency? If current tests for vitamin D levels say so, then how do we know that their bodies are not up-regulating the signaling effects of vitamin D somewhere else in the system? After all, when you factor out socioeconomic factors to rates of cancer among dark-skinned individuals, there's no evidence that they suffer from higher incidences of disease or more bone fractures. What other factors are at work when we observe an increase in cancer rates among African-Americans, for instance, living above the Mason-Dixon Line? On the other end of the spectrum, what about fair-skinned people who live closer to the equator? They can tan to provide more protection from the sun, but what about higher incidences of skin cancer?

The Surprising Truth about Skin Color

It turns out that the plot thickens more. The ability to tan is a trait that evolved several times throughout our evolution. We had to learn to survive not only in various regions of the globe, but we further had to develop ways to offset wild fluctuations in the sun's intensity from season to season. Research published in 2010 in the *Proceedings of the National Academy of Sciences* came to a convincing conclusion about people living in midlatitude regions such as China and the Mediterranean. If inhabitants of these regions had consistently dark skin, which blocks sunlight, then they wouldn't have produced enough vitamin D in the winter. Conversely, if they consistently had light skin, their bodies would have suffered another challenge: they would have been robbed of folate, a light-sensitive vitamin essential for cell division and repair. This is the same vitamin that women are told to consume prior to becoming pregnant and during pregnancy, as too little of it can lead to birth defects. (Synthetic folate used in prenatal supplements is folic acid.) Perhaps the biggest surprise of all in this latest study's findings is that the researchers postulate that sun-induced folate deficiency—not protection against things such as skin cancer—was the driving force behind the evolution of dark skin and tanning.

Which begs the question, why wouldn't tanning be evolution's solution to getting too much cancer-causing ultraviolet radiation? Or too much vitamin D, in addition to a bad sunburn? For starters, you can't overdose on vitamin D through sunlight, so we can throw out that idea. The body, not surprisingly, regulates the amount required so there's never any excess vitamin D circulating in the bloodstream. Lifeguards, for example, are famous for boasting levels of vitamin D that are more than five times greater than that of the general population, and you don't hear about them falling victim to toxic levels of D. (You can, however, overdose on supplemental vitamin D; it takes a lot, somewhere in the ballpark of repeated megadoses of more than 10,000 IU per day, but it can happen and requires medical attention.) Your body has a huge capacity to make vitamin D at any age from UVB sources. While aging does decreases levels of the provitamin D molecule responsible for making vitamin D in the skin, your body still has enough ingredients to make adequate vitamin D with adequate amounts of sunshine even when you are ninety years old.

If tanning has nothing to do with preventing vitamin D over-load, then what is it for? The answer illustrates another beautiful way in which the body maintains an intricate system designed to prevent imbalances that cause harm . . . and to perpetuate life.

Survival of the Fittest

You may not have noticed a little fact that I just mentioned and that has everything to do with survival of the fittest. Evolution doesn't care whether you suffer from skin cancer. Sunburn and most skin cancers do not alter your ability to procreate, so they are not selection factors. Destroying precious folate that's needed to produce healthy children, on the other hand, is something that evolution will protect.

It's not a coincidence that most cancers emerge after our child-bearing years. In the fourth and fifth decade of life, evolution doesn't have much interest in protecting us anymore because we're less likely to have—or be able to bear—children. Most of us lose nature's policing, if you will, once we reach middle age. It's also worth pointing out that nature doesn't necessarily care what gene you have that dictates your skin color. Lots of genetic variables can result in light, or conversely dark, skin. All nature is concerned with is that you can maintain your system in a way that will support future life. When light-skinned people use sunscreen to protect their skin, they are in effect protecting how they are genetically designed to look. When they tan in their environment, nature is doing what she does best: safeguarding an individual's fitness to procreate by preserving folate (and perhaps other things that we haven't yet identified).

We've only just begun to understand the changes that go on in the system when we make it "over the hill" and Mother Nature is no longer guarding our health as she did before. Now that people are living decades past their childbearing years, it's no wonder we see a higher prevalence of cancer and age-related disease. Mother Nature may be well-intentioned and good-spirited, but she is neither stupid nor overly gracious. She won't waste her energy on old dogs. We're left to our own devices once our bodies can no longer physiologically produce new life.

Furthermore, that the body can in no way overdose on vitamin D created through sunlight, as it can through supplementation, gives us a clue. We've perfected this clever process through millions of years and I think that speaks volumes on how we should obtain much of our vitamin D. Mother Nature proves her smarts again, for the sun is an excellent choice in guaranteeing that all vertebrates and humans get an essential vitamin.

Another clue to consider when you're reaching for that pill bottle:

vitamin D made in the skin lasts at least twice as long in the blood as vitamin D ingested from the diet. When you are exposed to sunlight, you not only make vitamin D but also at least five and up to ten different additional photoproducts that you would never get from dietary sources or from a supplement. The obvious question is, why would Mother Nature be making all of these vitamin D photoproducts if they weren't having a biologic effect? My guess is all of these photoproducts serve in the healthy functioning of our body's network, and future research will bear this out.

So How Much Do We Really Need?

By now you're probably confused as to whether you should be supplementing. Before I get to that answer, I must add more details to the vitamin D story. Recall earlier I hinted that not everyone's vitamin D receptors work exactly the same way. My receptors for vitamin D could be binding this molecule more tightly (or, for that matter, less tightly) than yours, thus affecting the total amount I need in my bloodstream. Researchers have proven that each of us has a genetic disposition to maintain a certain level of vitamin D, and that no number is perfect for everyone.

In June 2010, the *Lancet* published a large study showing that at least three, and probably four, genes contribute to the variability of vitamin D levels in the population. Just as eye color and blood types vary across the population—what we call in biology polymorphisms (more than one form or morph of the same thing)—vitamin D status varies. Interestingly, worldwide, vitamin D is at a mean concentration of about 20 ng/mL with little variation between countries (which by today's standards is considered "deficient"). What's more interesting is that there's much greater variation *within* countries, from lower than 8 to 80 ng/mL and higher. Such a wide variation cannot be explained, then, on just geography, since people who live at the same latitude are exposed to a relatively equal amount of vitamin D–generating UVB. Something more is going on within people's complex systems.

The researchers of this latest study pose a good question: Do the genes that control your vitamin D status also affect your body's response to vitamin D supplementation? If so, should this be taken into account when considering artificial intake of vitamin D through supplementation? All of this begs a more obvious question: What does it mean to be "deficient" or "insufficient"? How can anyone know exactly what "deficient" means to him or her? What are ideal levels? More to the point, who decides what is a "normal" vitamin D level? Unfortunately, human beings didn't arrive on Earth with an instruction manual defining our normal function!

I hope that you're not feeling unintelligent or hopelessly confused over all the fuzziness on this topic. Even the so-called experts in this field have wrestled with clarifying recommendations—equally confused by competing information and no doubt competing interests, as well. Adding insult to injury, yet another expert panel announced in late 2010 that taking high levels of vitamin D through supplements is unnecessary and could be harmful. It also concluded that calcium supplements are not needed. The fourteen-member committee was convened by the Institute of Medicine, an independent, nonprofit scientific body, at the request of the US and Canadian governments. It was asked to examine the available data—nearly one thousand publications—to determine how much vitamin D and calcium people were getting, how much was needed for optimal health, and how much was too much. The group said most people have adequate amounts of vitamin D in their blood supplied by their diets and natural sources such as sunshine, and that *for most people*, taking extra calcium and vitamin D supplements is not warranted.

This isn't to say that vitamin D supplementation is never justified. *For most people* is the key term here. In some instances perhaps a person should consider supplementing. People who avoid the sun, lather up with sunscreen on a cold winter's day, and don't eat any foods rich in vitamin D such as cold-water fish may want to consider supplementing. But acknowledge that the data have yet to show this is necessary, and you may not need as much as you think. This recent panel also concluded that 600 IU a day is plenty. You'll end up getting more than enough just in casual sun exposure and through fortified foods such as milk, juice, cereal, and even some mushrooms.

Keep in mind, though, that we have no way of knowing what effect vitamin D from supplemental sources could be having on other nodes in our network. As I hope I've made clear throughout this book, the notion that "this is good for everybody" doesn't make sense. When you affect one node, you don't know what it's doing downstream. So you don't know what changes all that extra vitamin D is doing to your receptors and their internal feedback loops, which drive your body's homeostasis.

The Magic of Our Body's Built-in Technology

Our bodies are equipped with some remarkable technology that would stump even the brightest engineers charged with trying to copy it in any man-made machine. I've been using the term *receptor* with regard to vitamin D but haven't fully defined what receptors are biochemically. Of all the biological concepts that a layperson would do well to understand, this is one of them. You likely learned about receptors in high school but have since long forgotten about them. They are not just related to vitamin D, but also explain how they work through the lens of the vitamin D story once again allows me to make a few points. Having a rough grasp of how receptors function can go a long way in helping you rethink exactly what it means to change your natural system through such things as vitamins and supplements.

A receptor is a protein molecule that's embedded in either the plasma membrane or the cytoplasm of a cell. It's what facilitates the physical attachments of other proteins or molecules to the cell so they can have an intended effect. These other molecules, which signal change in the cell, and hence are called signaling molecules, can be neurotransmitters, hormones, pharmaceutical drugs, or toxins. Our cells maintain receptors for different molecules, and virtually all of our cells and tissues contain receptors specifically designed for vitamin D. Here's the important point: a cell can increase or decrease the number of receptors to a given molecule, such as vitamin D, to alter its sensitivity to this molecule. Cells do this all the time to maintain that beautiful overall homeostasis. When they increase the number of receptors, we call that up-regulation. Conversely, when cells decrease the number of receptors to become less sensitive to a certain molecule, we call that down-regulation. This balancing act between up-regulation and down-regulation is the heart and soul of our homeostatic patterns. When there's too much of one thing, we down-regulate; and when there's not enough of another, we up-regulate. In economics, we call this the law of supply and demand. By way of example, take a look at the following figures:

Vitamin D Supplementation

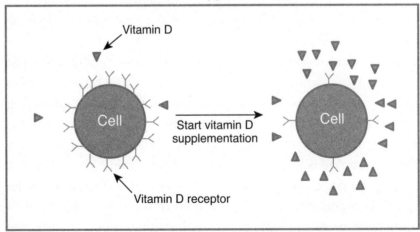

When your cells are deluged with vitamin D (as they are on the cell to the right), they will pull back on their sensitivity to vitamin D by reducing their number of receptors for vitamin D. But if there's a perceived shortfall of vitamin D in the bloodstream, your cells will up-regulate—create more receptors for vitamin D—to become more sensitive to every vitamin D molecule that passes by.

What happens, then, when we consume lots of vitamin D from unnatural sources such as supplements? (I use the term *unnatural* to imply that it's not coming from the sun, which is a source of vitamin D that has built-in regulatory mechanisms.) No doubt our bodies are adept at adjusting using their feedback loops as I just described, and the constant surplus of vitamin D means our cells are constantly down-regulating. If we took the supplemental vitamin D away, our cells would up-regulate to make up the difference.

Vitamin D has multiple downstream signaling molecules, for the vitamin D receptor signals several reactions. For this reason, changing one part of that signaling system may not mean much. We don't yet have a way of measuring functional vitamin D status, we just have a way of measuring one node. So when you receive your test results back indicating that you are low in vitamin D, are you really low in vitamin D signaling or vitamin D activity? As surprising as this may sound, there's no way to know using current technology and our library of medical wisdom. It's like looking at a stock and asking yourself if you should buy it based on a single piece of information. Consider this: If someone tells you that Coke has $8.2 billion in sales annually, should you pick up a few more shares of its stocks to add to your portfolio? Knowing Coke's sales figures is an interesting data point, but it doesn't tell the whole story. What if Coke is swimming in debt and has a terrible price-to-earnings ratio? Coke may have just ramped up advertising dramatically to increase sales, but profits may have plummeted due to the increased expenses. Even if you don't understand the significance of these financial terms in investment-speak, it's a good analogy because the body has its own set of arcane terms we're only just beginning to comprehend. And in the vitamin D language, we just don't know yet how to define true vitamin D deficiency, insufficiency, or other variations. Just as you could buy the stock, you could also take the pill, but you might be doing yourself damage down the road.

This doesn't mean that you will fail in your attempts to be healthy should you choose to focus on a single node and take a pill to address that node. We may want to attend to the pros and cons for addressing lots of nodes, as well as make some compromises. But I want you to be aware that a single node does not adequately represent the complex network. With more than 75 percent of individuals in the United States vitamin D deficient, and over 97 percent of African-Americans in the United States deficient, but with age-adjusted hip-fracture incidence notably *declining* over the last two decades, one has to wonder, where is the disconnect?

In my opinion, vitamin D cannot explain all the gaps and contradictions in the story. Before we make grand leaps and wild claims about its potential benefits, we must conduct further tests and push for refinements to our current measuring methods.

What About Other "Drugs"?

The lively deliberations over vitamin D will continue, and the overall discussion it instigates is useful. It makes a plausible case against overly general recommendations for everyone regardless of their vitamin D (or fill in the blank) status using current testing technology. It also adds caution where caution is warranted, because I don't believe that downing thousands of units of vitamin D through a supplement is what the body likes. Anything that artificially changes the body's system can be considered a drug, so, yes, we can and should call vitamins drugs. They meddle with the body's inherent homeostatic controls and thus might interrupt certain processes and ultimately have harmful effects that we cannot measure yet using current technology.

I often find myself in the center of heated conversations at dinner parties among those who devote an entire drawer in their kitchen or bathroom to bottles and vials of multivitamins and other supplements. When we're exposed daily to marketing ploys telling us to consume more antioxidants, vitamins, and other processed nutrients, it can be hard to ask the tough questions—especially when they go against everything we've been taught and led to believe.

Health Rule

Be wary of headlines that tell you what's good or bad for you. Scrutinize data before accepting it as dogma.

7

The Truth About Synthetic Shortcuts

*How to Save Hundreds of Dollars a Year and
Rethink the Need for Supplements and Vitamins*

I f ever there was a book that transported me back to an era that
longed for medical breakthroughs, it was James Lind's *A Treatise
of the Scurvy*, which was published in 1753. Interestingly, as history would have it, Lind's writings would come to inform some of
my most important research in modern times.

During the eighteenth century, entire wars were decided not
by weapons or manpower, but by the diets of the soldiers. Scurvy
killed more British sailors than enemy action, and it helped cost
the French the Battle of Trafalgar. Of all the disaster stories about
scurvy, none received more fanfare in Europe than that of George
Anson's catastrophic attempt to circumnavigate the world between
1740 and 1742. Within the first ten months Anson lost nearly two-
thirds of his crew (thirteen hundred out of two thousand) to the
disease. Then, during the Seven Years' War between 1756 and 1763,

the Royal Navy reported that it conscripted 184,899 sailors, of whom 133,708 died of disease or were "missing," and scurvy was the principal disease.

James Lind would go down in history as one of the first to try to understand scurvy. A Scottish military doctor for the Royal Navy, Lind made prescient recommendations to bring fresh limes on board ships going to sea, which is what gave the British sailors the nickname "Limeys." Lind had a hunch that lime juice could prevent scurvy. He was close in his predictions, but it didn't always work. When Lind autopsied the ravaged bodies of people who had died at sea from the malady, he came across some confusing findings that would preoccupy the better part of his life. In his historic 1753 *Treatise*, Lind wrote, "What was very surprising, the brains of those poor creatures were always sound and entire." He struggled immensely to come to grips with precisely what caused scurvy and how it could be eradicated.

Scurvy is a hellish disease that we now know is caused by a deficiency of vitamin C, but in Lind's day, the concept of vitamins was unknown and would be for a couple more centuries. (Scurvy was thought to be an infectious disease far into the twentieth century.) Vitamin C serves multiple purposes in the body, from its role in the manufacture of the neurotransmitter norepinephrine to aiding in fat metabolism, collagen synthesis, and iron absorption. During evolution, humans—along with a few other species—lost the gene that would allow us to make our own vitamin C in the liver (the mouse, surprisingly, still possesses the vitamin C synthesis gene). So, lacking vitamin C has dire consequences, scurvy being chief among them. Without vitamin C to keep the body's "scaffolding" together, its connective tissue begins to degrade and fall apart. Scurvy leads to the formation of spots on the skin, spongy gums, and bleeding from the mucous membranes. The spots are most abundant on the thighs and legs, and a person with the ailment looks pale, feels depressed, and is partially immobilized. Advanced scurvy leads to open, suppurating wounds and loss of teeth. Eventually death occurs as the body continues to break down.

Although Lind was not the first to suggest citrus fruit as a remedy for scurvy, he was the first to study their effect by a systematic experiment he conducted in 1747. It ranks as one of the first clinical trials in the history of medicine. Lind would be memorialized in medicine for more than just suggesting that the secret to preventing scurvy rested in oranges and lemons. He became a pioneer of naval hygiene in the Royal Navy, and he argued for the health benefits of better ventilation aboard naval ships, the improved cleanliness of sailors' bodies, clothing, and bedding, and belowdecks fumigation with sulfur and arsenic. He also proposed that freshwater could be obtained by distilling seawater. His work advanced the practice of preventive medicine and improved nutrition.

But he never understood the root cause of the disease that devastated sailors and explorers of his era. His grand treatise was virtually ignored. Lind, like most of the medical establishment at the time, believed that scurvy was a result of ill-digested and putrefying food within the body, bad water, excessive work, and living in a damp atmosphere that prevented healthful perspiration. Thus, while he recognized the benefits of citrus fruit, he never advocated citrus juice as a single solution. He believed that scurvy had multiple causes, which therefore required multiple remedies. In all fairness, not all was lost given his inability to decisively settle the causes and the treatment of scurvy. Lind's writings established his overarching theory of the disease and showed what part diet, and in particular fruit and vegetables, played in this theory. His treatise offered a glimmer of truth to what constitutes a healthy diet, of which fruits and vegetables are key.

In 1762 Lind penned an essay on the most effective means of preserving the health of seamen. In it he recommended growing salad—i.e., watercress (662 mg vitamin C per 100 g)—on wet blankets. This was actually put in practice, and in the winter of 1775 the British army in North America was supplied with mustard and cress seeds. Had Lind been able to pinpoint the root cause of scurvy—a lack of vitamin C—he could probably have saved a lot more sailors than through a long list of helpful recommendations. When he performed those autopsies, he must have felt something or someone was conspiring against him and his fellow men. As he commented in his *Treatise*, how could the brains of scurvy patients be so beautifully preserved and disease-free? It didn't make sense, and it would take science a long time to fully understand this disease.

Your Brain, and Tumors, on Vitamin C

Let's flash forward a few hundred years to 1996 when I was at Memorial Sloan-Kettering Cancer Center in New York working in the laboratory of David Golde, M.D., who was physician in chief at the time. We were trying to pick up where Lind had left off. Okay, so that may be a little bit of an exaggeration, because what my colleagues and I found haphazardly happened to help explain the minor medical mystery that Lind had observed among those autopsies. But we weren't studying scurvy or how vitamin C reaches the brain. We were trying to figure out how cancer tumors are able to gorge themselves at the expense of the surrounding normal tissue, so we decided to trail vitamin C as it traveled through the body.

Many great leaps in science have been made when alert people, looking for something else, came across a major discovery and recognized its importance. Our discovery was no exception. In our experiment, we injected the tail veins of mice with a version of vitamin C that would glow as it was absorbed in the body. Much to our surprise, none of it went into the brain.

The brain has a spectacular defense network known as the blood-brain barrier, which selects the chemicals that can enter and leave. In some cases, it is far easier to drill holes in the skull and drop drugs onto the surface than to send them past the blood-brain barrier.

Doctors resort to this technique when they need to administer certain drugs to treat brain-related disease or brain cancer, although the structure of the blood-brain barrier makes even this difficult. The marvels of modern medicine allowed us to take this experiment further and ultimately determine that the brain is quite clever when it comes to absorbing vitamin C. It doesn't actually let vitamin C in—it permits an altered version of vitamin C called dehydroascorbic acid to sneak past its gatekeeper, the blood-brain barrier. This is actually how vitamin C gets into all of your tissues in the body, but because the brain contains more of these special transporters, vitamin C levels are ten times higher in the central nervous system than elsewhere in the body. The brain can hoard the vitamin C that the body takes in from external sources. Regulation of vitamin C in the brain is essential as it's needed to produce the neurotransmitter norepinephrine.

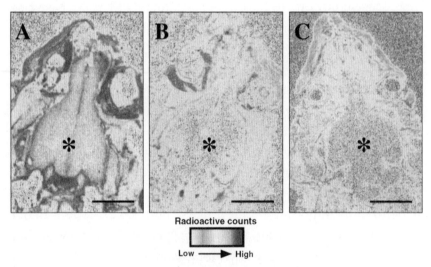

The picture above is of three brain digital scans of a rat with A) radioactive-labeled ascorbic acid (vitamin C in its natural reduced form and not transportable), B) radioactive-labeled dehydroascorbic acid (the oxidized form and transportable), and C) radioactive-labeled sucrose (a sugar molecule that is not transportable). Source: JCI 1997; 100(11):2842–2848.

To get a picture of the process, think of an open umbrella that can't fit through a narrow doorway. But if you close the umbrella and change its shape, it will slip right through the door. Once on the other side, you can reopen the umbrella. That's what happens to vitamin C. The brain has a tight doorway that permits ascorbic acid (the chemical name for vitamin C) to enter only in its oxidized form (called dehydroascorbic acid), which is slightly different from the molecules in your orange juice. Once inside the brain, the oxidized ascorbic acid changes back to its original form. We cannot just ingest dehydroascorbic acid because it's too unstable.

Vitamin C is essential to keep the central nervous system functioning properly, and it uses the same transport mechanism that the brain employs to ferry glucose across its formidable border. Lind's autopsied brains were fine because they had their own stash of vitamin C, which the rest of the body lacked. This ensures that the brain would be the last organ depleted of vitamin C. So if you want to send extra vitamin C to the brain, popping tablets is a waste, because most of it will be passed in the urine, and little of it will get to the brain.

Ascorbic Acid

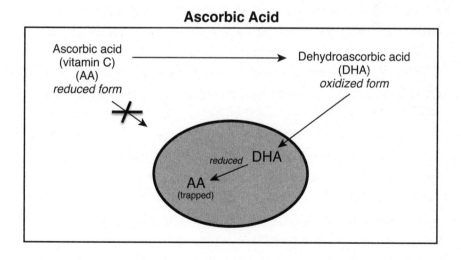

Can we force-feed ascorbic acid to the brain? Certainly, using the altered version of the vitamin. Manipulating vitamin C levels in the brain may turn out to be helpful in combating all sorts of neurological disorders. Vitamin C is an antioxidant, a little Pac-Man molecule that chews up dangerous chemicals known as oxidants, or free radicals. The oxidants are regarded as the rogue bullets in many diseases, injuring the cells at a genetic level. Oxidants are linked to Alzheimer's and Parkinson's diseases, and also to the brain damage that occurs when a person suffers a stroke. They are also known to be players in the general aging, hence their infamy in antiaging circles, and the popularity of antioxidants. I have to caution that this system of oxidation is not that simple, though, as we'll see later in this book.

Our little experiment has led to new trials that seek to understand vitamin C's, and its derivatives', use as drugs to help mop up free radicals in the brain that could be injurious and responsible for exacerbating brain disease. But we wouldn't necessarily want to do this for brain cancer or any other type of cancer. Although vitamin C might help prevent cancer, it can become an archenemy once you're cancering because tumors enjoy vitamin C. They devour vitamin C like candy, so you could be feeding your cancer rather than fighting it if you consume excess vitamin C. In the late 1990s, I was also part of David Golde's team at Memorial Sloan-Kettering Cancer Center that discovered that cancer tumors feast on large amounts of vitamin C. They do so by hitching a ride through the same physical pathway that glucose takes to cross the cell membrane and into the cell. Malignant cells engulf more glucose than normal cells to obtain the energy they need to grow excessively and gobble up more vitamin C, too.

Tumors are famous for having lots of inflammatory tissue around them as well as large numbers of these transporters for glucose and vitamin C. The cancer cells are dividing and hence need glucose, which up-regulates these transporters. Cancers grow quickly, many times outgrowing their own blood supply and oxygen, which explains why there is necrotic or dead tissue in the cancer area—triggering inflammation. Vitamin C is always in our bloodstream, but it only enters cells when it's oxidized to dehydroascorbic acid. The vitamin C (ascorbic acid) from the blood will be oxidized right at the local tumor site due to all the inflammatory molecules at the tumor, then slip into the tumor, where it will be transformed back to ascorbic acid and trapped there for use by the cancerous cell to grow. Much of the anticancer therapy we use, namely radiation and chemotherapy, kills cells by creating free radicals (i.e., promoting oxidation). Thus, high concentrations of vitamin C, which acts mainly as an antioxidant, will inhibit these agents from their maximum cell kill. The cancer loves the vitamins and will use them for its own benefit—the growth I mentioned above.

To better grasp how vitamins in general work, and how they can become accomplices to cancerous growth, it helps to understand what a vitamin is exactly, and how they can have "antioxidant" properties.

Synthetic Shortcuts

The term *vitamin* was derived from *vitamine*, a word invented by Polish scientist Casimir Funk, who combined *vital* and *amine* to create "amine of life." The word *amine* refers to a specific chemical compound containing nitrogen that was thought to be responsible for preventing beriberi, a disease caused by vitamin B deficiency and perhaps other similar dietary-deficiency diseases. Amine proved not to be the lifesaving compound scientists thought it was, but the word, which was shorted to *vitamin*, stuck.

Vitamins are organic compounds (i.e., they contain carbon) that team up with proteins in the body chiefly to create enzymes that work to regulate the body's functionality. We cannot create enough of our requisite vitamins physiologically, but they are easy to obtain through diet. Most vitamin supplements on the market today are called multivitamins. Obviously, this means that they contain multiple vitamins, thirteen of which have been identified as needed by the body to function well: vitamin A, eight kinds of vitamin B (thiamin, riboflavin, niacin, pantothenic acid, B6, B12, folacin, and biotin), vitamin C, vitamin D, vitamin E, and vitamin K. Virtually all multivitamins contain vitamins in doses that are several orders of magnitude larger than what you need to prevent any deficiency-related ailment. For example, 30 milligrams a day will prevent scurvy, which is what's found in half of an orange. Some multivitamins, however, will stock a whopping 1,000 milligrams of vitamin C.

About half of US adults, maybe more, take vitamins and other dietary supplements, spending over $25 billion yearly on dietary supplements, so I can only imagine what the average annual expense is for someone who takes multivitamins and supplements regularly. Just as we haven't had clinical vitamin D deficiency disease—characterized by bone ailments such as rickets and osteomalacia—in this country for decades, we haven't experienced any other types of vitamin-deficiency disease other than outlier cases that have unique circumstances or causes and that don't reflect trends in the general population. Scurvy is extremely rare, and when it happens, it's among patients who are elderly or alcoholic and who subsist on diets devoid of fresh fruits and vegetables.

I have no problem with people taking vitamins to correct a bona fide deficiency or to address certain conditions, such as pregnancy. Women contemplating pregnancy or who are already pregnant, especially in the early months, should speak with their doctor about taking a prescribed prenatal vitamin. Even though prenatal vitamins are available over the counter, I recommend the prescribed ones because they pass stricter quality controls so you know that you're getting what's on the label. But for the rest of us who aren't in those unique circumstances, taking vitamins generically for health makes no sense. A vitamin is something that the body cannot synthesize, and we can get all the vitamins we need from the foods we eat, assuming that you make an effort to eat nutrient-dense foods from natural sources. More vitamins doesn't mean better. Although the argument has been made for "topping off" our vitamin intake by supplementing with multivitamins—to help make up for any shortages due to a less-than-ideal diet—I cannot justify this as a rational approach. Michael Pollan stated it brilliantly when he wrote in his book *In Defense of Food*, "That anyone should need to write a book advising people to 'eat food' could be taken as a measure of our alienation and confusion."

Indeed, Pollan nails it on the head. Why, in this age of plenty, do we need to rely on manufactured pills to get our vitamins and other nutrients? Why are we so out of touch with our own reality? One of the main reasons we are estranged from real meals today that are close to nature is because fast and processed foods abound. Another is we are led to believe that we will be healthier and feel better if we boost our intake of vitamins and nutrients through pills, powders, elixirs, juices, and the like. *Antioxidant* in particular has become a buzzword of the boomer generation, and antioxidant products, alongside other formulas such as resveratrol, which promise to reverse all the signs and symptoms of aging, are marketed today as though they represent the fountain of youth. Ironically, it is estimated that one-third of adults in high-income countries (which means that they have access to the best, most nutrient-dense foods that money can buy) consume antioxidant supplements. But what, if anything, does taking antioxidant supplements really do? The answer might surprise you.

The Anti of Antioxidants

Let's return for a moment to this idea of an antioxidant. By definition, an antioxidant is a substance that is capable of "blocking" the effects of oxidation. Oxidation, to be clear, is a normal biological process. Oxidation happens everywhere in nature, as well as in our bodies. It occurs during the natural process of metabolism, which is simply the body's way of turning calories (energy) from food and oxygen from the air into energy that can be used by the body. Oxidation is very much a part of our being, but when it begins to run amok or there's too much oxidation without a balance of antioxidant action, it can become harmful. "Oxidation" of course entails oxygen, but not the kind we breathe. The form of oxygen that's involved here is simply O because it's not paired with another oxygen molecule (O_2). Although the word *oxidation* is often couched in negative terms, it's really just a chemical reaction that takes place constantly in our bodies to sustain its health and life through certain biological processes. It can support reactions that contribute to our health as much as it can perpetuate reactions that cause harm.

It might help to think of oxidation as a combustion process, and the exhaust is made up of by-products called free radicals (or, more technically, reactive oxygen species, or ROS for short). Free radicals were first identified by Moses Gomberg at the University of Michigan in 1900. They are molecules that have lost an electron. Normally electrons spin around in pairs, but forces such as stress, pollution, ultraviolet light from the sun, and ordinary bodily activities (even breathing) can make one of them break off. When that happens, the molecule starts ricocheting around, trying to steal electrons from other molecules. This commotion is the oxidation, a chain of events that attacks cells and, as we'll see in chapter 9, kicks off inflammation, which creates more free radicals. Oxidation is a necessary evil in the body's attempts to conduct reactions and to support its overall homeostasis. Free radicals are necessary for living organisms: in addition to being normal by-products of critical biological processes, they are used by our immune system (the granulocytes and macrophages) to kill bacteria, and they also act as part of the cell signaling process for many "normal" functions of the cell.

But when the oxidation is in overdrive, which results in a surfeit of free radicals, problems can emerge. Much in the way inflammation promotes healing but can become dangerously chronic, so too can oxidation. Because oxidized tissues, cells, proteins, and DNA harmed by free radicals don't function normally, many scientists have hypothesized that uncontrolled oxidation in the body leads to a host of health challenges, from wrinkles and low metabolism to obesity, heart disease, cancer, dementia, and other diseases and signs of aging. If the health foods and supplements industry is to be believed, antioxidants are the panacea of modern times. Until the word *antioxidant* became part of the common vernacular thanks to the antiaging industry, it was hard to sell people on the benefits of fruits and vegetables, but now we can ascribe many of the health pluses of produce to their antioxidant ingredients that will shield us from oxidative stress.

Not surprisingly, the body has its own way of keeping free radicals in check. It harbors a store of enzymes that can neutralize free radicals, including glutathione reductase, glutathione peroxidase, catalase, and superoxide dismutase, as well as chemicals such as bilirubin and uric acid. Vitamins we can easily obtain in our diets such as vitamins A, C, and E can also help in this regard. They act as Good Samaritans by gladly donating electrons to free radicals, which interrupts the oxidative chain reaction and helps prevent the damage these loose cannons do.

What happens, then, when we consume excess free radicals

> If you look at all the vitamin studies done on more than a thousand people in the last few decades, almost all of them have shown an increased risk of cancer. Some of these results were statistical, but some were not. The body likes to create free radicals to attack bad cells, including cancerous ones. If you block that mechanism by taking copious vitamins, especially those touted as antioxidants, you block your body's natural ability to control itself. You block a physiological process. You disrupt a system we don't fully understand yet.

through vitamins and the like that the body doesn't need? Can that in any way disrupt the body's normal balancing act between creating free radicals to attack bad cells, some of which could be cancerous, and corralling and neutralizing free radicals that can get out of control? If you upset that delicate balancing act, you block a physiological process and you disrupt a system that we don't yet fully understand. Perhaps this is why, based on the review of numerous studies, the evidence for taking vitamins just doesn't live up to all the hype.

Lots of Hype, Little Indisputable Data

If you're like most health-conscious Americans, multivitamins have been a key part of your daily routine, or you at least think about it daily and do your best to remember to take them. As recently as 2002, no less an authority than the *Journal of the American Medical Association* recommended that "all adults take one multivitamin daily." Your doctor likely endorsed this recommendation, too. But today, a tsunami of scientific data has resulted in a reversal in thinking among many experts in the health and nutrition community, myself included. To look at the multivitamin as an insurance policy is like looking at a marriage license as a guarantee of the union's permanence. It is, quite frankly, naive and overly trusting.

Little data, if any, shows that ingesting more vitamins or antioxidants benefits health or changes the effects of free radicals in the body. I am not aware of any clinical trial demonstrating a general health benefit to taking supplemental vitamins and have in fact come across some disturbing negative effects found in some studies. But I've also found that studies tend to conflict so much with one another as to be meaningless. I believe that this harkens back to the original premise of the book: the body is a complex system. Changing one variable will have many effects in the system that we have yet to develop technology to fully comprehend. Increased ingestion of antioxidants may push the system in the "wrong" direction. Before I even get to the mix of studies done on some of these perceived health promoters, let me first play devil's advocate and expose one such study that put a new spin on things, demonstrating that not all antioxidants are as wildly helpful as they seem. They can inhibit oxidation in a way that has detrimental, as opposed to health-enhancing, effects.

In 2009, researchers at the University of Cardiff in Wales showed that vitamin C has a "pro-oxidant" alter ego that can benefit arteries by increasing the production of free radicals. Their study, which was published in the journal *Cardiovascular Research*, revealed a surprising new look at why vitamin C helps patients with cardiovascular challenges. As Sam Wong of the British Heart Foundation perfectly described it in an article for *The Guardian* that year (and who aptly characterized vitamin C as having an "alter ego"), the layer of smooth muscle that envelops our arteries is often unable to relax in patients with high blood pressure, high cholesterol, diabetes, and heart failure. Consequently, the vessels stay tightly constricted, increasing strain on the heart. Injections of vitamin C can help the arteries to relax, an effect that has been attributed to an increased production of nitric oxide, which is an important vessel-relaxing signal molecule.

But the Cardiff team discovered that something else was happening independently of nitric oxide. Vitamin C reacts with dissolved oxygen to generate hydrogen peroxide, a potentially harmful unstable chemical. However, hydrogen peroxide can also increase the strength of electrical signals from the blood vessel's lining, telling the surrounding muscle to relax. This led the researchers to shed a more positive light on oxidants that our body might need to conduct healthy physiological functioning. The catch, of course, is finding the balance, which is something that the Cardiff researchers were clear to point out. Too many oxidative molecules can hurt, as can too little. Future therapies might have to strike a balance between promoting and suppressing oxidative stress.

Fair warning: If you're thinking of downing vitamin C in the hopes of protecting your arteries, bear in mind that large clinical trials have found vitamin C supplements to be completely ineffective at preventing cardiovascular disease. This is probably because high blood concentrations of vitamin C get quickly filtered out by your kidneys.

The story doesn't end there, however. Tetrahydrobiopterin, another pro-oxidant the Cardiff team examined, has shown some promise in trials for reducing blood pressure when taken orally. In the future, doctors might one day prescribe pro-oxidants to treat vascular diseases. But again, there's no doubt that producing unstable chemicals in excess can be harmful, as oxidative stress can also cause arteries to constrict, which is yet another reason to find the balance. Many variables are at play and we don't currently understand all of them.

Over the years, many studies have been done to explore the role that antioxidants may have in heart disease, and, more specifically, the potential link between the oxidation of bad (LDL) cholesterol and antioxidants. This type of oxidation contributes to the buildup of fatty plaque on artery walls (atherosclerosis), which can eventually slow or block blood flow to the heart.

But little progress has been made in these studies; first, because the designs of some of them left their results open to question. For example, some of the studies used too few participants to obtain valid results. Some used doses of vitamins that were later thought too low. Some had a limited duration of treatment, and others could not determine whether the beneficial results were from the antioxidants or other lifestyle factors.

Aside from experiments designed to determine the benefits of a specific supplement, it's important to note that people who take vitamins and supplements tend to be healthier than the population at large, and their health probably has nothing to do with the supplements they take. It's well documented that vitamin takers tend to be leaner, more affluent, and more educated. They drink and smoke less; they exercise and go to the doctor more. They're healthy in ways that do not include their use of multivitamins. So, making any judgments about the advantages of taking supplements by studying just those who make a habit of it, or those who participate in studies that entail supplements, is somewhat useless. Studies to examine the benefits of any given supplement can be riddled with flaws. Furthermore, among the studies that have been well designed, their results have been less than straightforward, wildly differing from one another. Some found benefit in antioxidants. Some didn't. Still others found potential harm from one of the antioxidants, beta-carotene.

Surely you've come across a few of these conflicting reports, for the media has announced the findings of these contradictory studies with great fanfare. "Take vitamin E to fight heart disease." Or: "Don't take vitamin E because it increases your risk for heart failure." All of this leaves us disoriented about the best way to support our health. Similar headlines have attacked other vitamins and supplements with equally polarizing messages. Thankfully, sound research from some of our most trusted purveyors of medical wisdom has tried to put this uncertainty to rest. Today, the growing body of evidence—and scientific opinion held—is changing the landscape for these molecules.

For starters, researchers at the Cleveland Clinic attempted to clear up the confusion about supplement use by doing a meta-analysis—an overview study of the best-designed, largest studies of antioxidants. A meta-analysis is an excellent way to explore an idea because it allows investigators to combine the results of many studies, thereby allowing small benefits or harm to be seen that may not have been appreciated in any one study. The Cleveland group's findings were published in 2003 in the British medical journal the *Lancet*.

The researchers analyzed results from seven large, randomized trials of vitamin E, alone or in combination with other antioxidants, and eight of beta-carotene, which is a precursor of vitamin A. The doses of vitamin E ranged from 50–800 international units (IU);

for beta-carotene, the doses were 15–50 milligrams (mg). Overall, 81,788 patients were included in the vitamin E portion of the
meta-analysis and 138,113 in the beta-carotene portion. The researchers looked for the effect of these antioxidant vitamins on
death rates, either from cardiovascular disease or from any other
cause, what's referred to in scientific circles as "all-cause mortality."
Much to the their surprise, vitamin E did not provide any benefit
in lowering mortality compared to control treatments, and it did
not significantly decrease the risk of cardiovascular death or stroke
("cerebrovascular accident"). The lack of any beneficial effect was
seen consistently regardless of the doses of vitamins used and the
diversity of the patient populations. The researchers concluded that
their study did "not support the routine use of vitamin E."

On the other hand, beta-carotene led to a small but statistically
significant *increase* in death rates and a slight increase in cardiovascular death in particular. This led the Cleveland group to call their
findings "especially concerning" because beta-carotene doses are
commonly included in over-the-counter vitamin supplements and
multivitamin supplements that have been advocated for widespread
use. The researchers noted that using vitamin supplements that contain beta-carotene should be "actively discouraged" because of the
increase in the risk of death. They also recommended discontinuing
the study of beta-carotene supplements altogether because of their
potential danger.

On the heels of this study came another that made vitamin E
look as if it had a split personality. A researcher at Brigham and
Women's Hospital in Boston led an international team that analyzed
data from the medical literature. This group reviewed nine trials
published through January 2010 that included more than 118,000
participants; 59,357 took vitamin E supplements and 59,408 took a
placebo. The trials did not include people who took multivitamins.
Although the risk remained relatively small, the team found that
taking vitamin E supplements *increased* the risk of hemorrhagic

stroke, in which bleeding occurs in the brain. But vitamin E supplements *reduced* the risk of ischemic stroke, the more common type of stroke, in which blood flow to the brain is blocked. Confusing?

Perpetual Paradoxes

Paradoxical findings like these are common and underscore what I've been saying since the beginning of the book: when it comes to the intricate human body, you cannot do one thing to affect one thing. When you take a drug, it will affect your entire system, not just the targeted area you wish the drug to influence. More than anything else, these findings further strengthen the contention that diet supplements are no substitute for good eating habits, exercise, weight loss, and smoking cessation as a means of minimizing the risk of heart disease and stroke. Let's look at another comprehensive study of late, which pit the vitamin debate up against the subject of cancer.

In the Alpha-Tocopherol (a form of vitamin E), Beta-Carotene (ATBC) Cancer Prevention Study, the US National Cancer Institute teamed up with the National Institute for Health and Welfare of Finland from 1985 to 1993 to conduct a cancer prevention trial. The purpose of the study was to determine whether certain vitamin supplements would prevent lung cancer and other cancers in a group of 29,133 male smokers in Finland. The fifty- to sixty-nine-year-old participants took a pill daily for five to eight years that contained one of the following: 50 mg of vitamin E, 20 mg of beta-carotene, both, or a placebo. Vitamin E and beta-carotene were chosen because previous studies have linked high dietary intake and high serum levels of these micronutrients to a reduced risk of cancer, particularly lung cancer. Both are antioxidants, compounds that may prevent carcinogens from damaging DNA and other cellular systems.

The ATBC study was conducted in Finland because of the high

lung cancer rates in men in that country, which were due primarily to cigarette smoking. Furthermore, Finland had a clinic system for the screening and treatment of lung diseases, mainly tuberculosis, through which the recruited population of smokers could participate in the study. Finland also has a national cancer registry, which keeps track of all the cancer cases identified in that country, a vital measurement for the large trial. Finnish women were not included in the study because their rate of lung cancer was substantially lower than that for Finnish men. In 1985, the annual age-adjusted lung cancer rate for Finnish men was 67 cases per 100,000, and for women, 8 cases per 100,000.

The participants began taking the vitamin supplements in 1985 and stopped by April 1993. By then, beta-carotene's report card wasn't looking good: men who took it in supplement form had an 18 percent *increased* incidence of lung cancers and an 8 percent *increased* overall mortality. This outcome was unfortunately similar for those taking both beta-carotene and vitamin E. The verdict for vitamin E alone, however, wasn't so clear-cut. Vitamin E seemed to have no effect on lung cancer incidence or overall mortality, yet it showed signs of influencing other aspects of these people's health. There were 32 percent fewer cases of prostate cancer and 41 percent fewer deaths from prostate cancer among those taking the vitamin E alone. But there was a noticeable hitch: death from hemorrhagic stroke, which entails a lack of blood to the brain due to a ruptured blood vessel, *increased* by 50 percent in those taking vitamin E supplements, and especially among those with hypertension.

Luckily, the investigators here didn't lose interest in this unfolding story once their active trial ended in 1993. They kept a close watch on their participants for fourteen years thereafter, until December of 2007, using data from the national registries in Finland. They wanted to know more and produced some thought-provoking results:

- In the eight-year follow-up period, the group that had taken beta-carotene experienced a 7 percent higher overall death rate than men on the placebo. However, this elevation was largely limited to the first four to six years of follow-up; during the last two years, the overall death rates were comparable to people who did not receive beta-carotene. In the beta-carotene group, the higher death rate during the entire twenty-two year study was due to cardiovascular disease and lung cancer. The higher death rate during the active, eight-year supplementation period was due to cardiovascular disease alone.
- The increased risks for lung cancer that occurred in those who supplemented with beta-carotene began to fall soon after they stopped taking the vitamin and were similar to the placebo group within four years.
- The lower prostate cancer incidence rates in participants taking vitamin E supplements during the trial returned toward normal soon after the trial ended, but remained below the placebo group rates throughout the six-year postintervention period.

The adverse effects from beta-carotene and the beneficial effects from supplementation with vitamin E largely disappeared during the post-trial follow-up period. Really scrutinizing these findings, you'll notice a symmetry in the times during and after the trial. That is, the time it took for the elevated lung cancer rates and lower prostate cancer rates to happen was similar to the time for these adverse and beneficial effects to disappear. Once the trial ended, no additional beneficial effects on cancer or mortality were observed.

Clearly, the study shot down any upside to taking beta-carotene, and this has been confirmed in other large-scale prevention studies. One of the more famous of these, conducted in the United States, was the Beta-Carotene and Retinol Efficacy Trial (CARET), which compared the effects of beta-carotene plus vitamin A (in the form of retinyl palmitate) to placebo in 18,314 men and women ages forty-five to seventy-four who were either smokers, former smokers, and/or had been exposed to asbestos. A 28 percent higher lung cancer incidence and 17 percent higher overall mortality occurred in the group taking the vitamin supplementation.

As for vitamin E's potential benefits for preventing prostate cancer, the jury is still out. In 2007, when the National Institutes of Health–AARP Diet and Health Study was published, the results were convincing enough to further give people such as me pause in the use of supplements. This study investigated the association between multivitamin use, which typically contains vitamin E, and risk of prostate cancer in 295,344 men. All of the participants— aged fifty to seventy-one years old—were cancer free at enrollment in 1995 and 1996. During their five years of follow-up, 10,241 of these men were diagnosed with prostate cancer, among which 1,476 were advanced. To these researchers' surprise, those who admitted to taking lots of vitamins ("excessive use," defined as more than seven times per week) showed an *increased* risk of advanced and fatal prostate cancers. Although no association was observed between multivitamin use and the risk of treatable (early-stage) prostate cancer, the risk of fatal prostate cancer among those taking regular multivitamins was double!

Let me temper this result a bit before you jump to too many of your own conclusions. This NIH-AARP study that I just described was observational, and therefore potentially confounded by many other variables, but I will say that the sample studied was large, which reduced random errors, and that overall, the study was well conducted. The results are in accord with the results of systematic reviews and meta-analyses of randomized clinical trials. The findings lend further credence to the possibility of harm associated with increased use of supplements, including increased rates of cancer and death from cardiovascular problems. The study adds to the growing evidence that questions the beneficial value of antioxidant vitamin pills in generally well-nourished populations and underscores the possibility that antioxidant supplements could have unintended, and even negative, consequences for our health.

I could take up the next tens of pages of this book outlining similar studies that have further confirmed what I've long thought to be true: vitamins don't live up to the hype. But for fear of inundating you with too many academically minded summaries, let me briefly mention just a couple more that are more recent than those already described:

- In 2010, the Agency for Healthcare Research and Quality published a review of sixty-three randomized, controlled trials (again, the gold-standard research method) on multivitamins, finding that multivitamins did nothing to prevent cancer or heart disease in most populations. The only exception occurred in developing countries where nutritional deficiencies are widespread.
- In 2009, scientists at the Fred Hutchinson Cancer Research Center in Seattle, Washington, published a paper after following 160,000 postmenopausal women for about ten years. The researchers' conclusion: multivitamins failed to prevent cancer, heart disease, and all causes of death for all women they tracked—regardless of healthy eating habits.

Multivitamins aren't the only supplements that have been getting lots of press and unwarranted rave reviews. Selenium, a trace mineral that gets incorporated into proteins to make important antioxidants, has also gained popularity lately. But studies examining the benefits of selenium, especially with regard to warding off cancer, show that the mineral doesn't live up to the hype. Case in point: Between 2001 and 2004, more than thirty-five thousand men enrolled in the SELECT study (costing more than $130 million!), which stands for the *Sel*enium and Vitamin *E* *C*ancer Prevention *T*rial, a prevention clinical trial to see if one or both of these dietary supplements prevent prostate cancer. The trial, funded primarily by the National Cancer Institute (NCI), is being coordinated by the Southwest Oncology Group (SWOG), an international network of research institutions that receives NCI funding.

Although the participants are still being monitored today, they were told in October 2008 to stop taking their supplements. By then, the researchers had already determined a few things. For one, selenium and vitamin E, taken alone or together for an average of five and a half years, did not prevent prostate cancer. Secondly, some disturbing trends emerged that weren't statistically significant but nonetheless compelled researchers to sound alarms. Slightly more cases of prostate cancer occurred in men taking only vitamin E, and slightly more cases of diabetes in men taking only selenium. Why? We don't know. Neither of these findings proves an increased risk from the supplements and they could well be due to chance, but it's interesting to note nonetheless.

In the fall of 2011, a cautionary note was published in the *Journal of the American Medical Association* that further confirmed the SELECT study's bad report card for vitamin E. Although the original results didn't yield any statistically significant conclusions, over time it indeed became statistical: a 17 percent increased risk of prostate cancer was found among healthy men who took the vitamin E supplements. As the study authors state: "Given more than 50 percent of individuals 60 years or older are taking supplements containing vitamin E, and 23 percent of them are taking at least 400 IU/d despite a recommended daily dietary allowance of only 22.4 IU for adult men, the implications of our observations are substantial." The other issue is that the health implications of the supplements may not manifest for many years after the supplement is stopped.

All this once again supports the idea that changing a system, be it through supplementation or increasing one vitamin over another, can potentially have significant effects. Just as we cannot explain why some men taking selenium were at a higher risk of developing diabetes, we cannot expound on the complex network of how vitamins affect and alter our systems—for better or worse. It remains to be seen which vitamins could be worth taking by using new technologies that can help confirm how they can help or hinder health. For you, perhaps a daily dose of B complex could actually be beneficial to optimizing your system. Until you can know for sure, rest assured that all the studies to date on vitamins prove that they don't live up to their expensive billing.

Health Rule

Ditch shortcuts to nutrition and health, which can shortcut your life. Unless you are correcting a legitimate deficiency or addressing a condition such as pregnancy, then you likely don't need to be taking multivitamins and other supplements.

8

The Fallacy of "Fresh"

Hidden Dangers and Opportunities in Your Local Market

While it may seem presumptuous to entrust a multivitamin with the job of averting a heart attack or fending off cancerous growths in the body, in the back of our minds that's exactly what many of us are thinking. Or at least it's what we wish so badly to be true. Otherwise, why bother spending the money and swallowing all those pills? Or perhaps you do have lower expectations and just think that taking one would make you healthier in general by filling in gaps, lowering your risk for disease, improving your immunity, and increasing your energy level. We hear all the time that supplemental vitamins can do these things for us, but we forget to remember that these claims come mainly from the manufacturers and their savvy marketing departments. The scientific research on those benefits tells a different story, one that is especially discouraging for particular groups of people on which we'd expect vitamins to have a positive impact. A British review of eight studies, for instance, found zero evidence that multivitamins reduced infections in older adults. Among breast cancer patients undergoing radiation therapy, vitamins didn't improve fatigue. On the other end of the age spectrum, inner-city schoolchildren who took a multivitamin did not perform any better on tests or have fewer sick days than students who didn't take one. More disturbing still, a 2010 study of Swedish women revealed that those who took multivitamins were 19 percent more likely to be diagnosed with breast cancer over a ten-year period than those who didn't. Other research has linked excessive folic acid intake to higher colon cancer risk in people who are predisposed. Which begs the question, why would you accept even a tiny risk if you're not getting any benefit?

Unfortunately, our knowledge of the mechanisms of bioavailability, biotransformation, and the action of antioxidant supplements still has many deep gulfs. How many fruits and vegetables do we have to eat to obtain the perfect amount of these nutrients? Why is it not possible to take a vitamin pill to obtain the same effect as a balanced diet? One possibility is that supplements are factory processed and may not be safe compared with their naturally occurring counterparts. We now have a much better understanding of how well whole foods deliver their nutritional benefits and therefore know that the very concept of a multivitamin as a nutrient delivery system is limited. Consider that a typical multivitamin contains ten to twenty-five isolated nutrients, but fruits and vegetables have hundreds of active compounds with a long list of health properties. The vitamin C in a multivitamin is likely just not as effective as the vitamin C in a citrus fruit, where it's also surrounded by fiber and flavonoids and carotenoids (compounds found in plants that may have protective health benefits when consumed). The combined result of these nutrients working together is what really keeps you healthy.

Another possible explanation for the negative effects of antioxidant supplementation observed in trials is that the studies were conducted in middle- and high-income countries among populations already well saturated with vitamins and trace elements. We eat a pretty good diet, and as I've already stated, it's rare to see vitamin deficiency in this country. The typical American diet, despite our penchant for too much fat, sugar, and processed foods, provides 120 percent of the recommended dietary allowances for beta-carotene, vitamin A, and vitamin C, and dietary vitamin E deficiency has never been reported in the United States.

Something else to consider in light of this debate over the benefits of antioxidants is whether oxidative stress is a primary cause of chronic diseases and the aging or merely a consequence. I've raised this question before, and it begs to be reiterated: Is it helpful or harmful to artificially modulate the delicate balance between oxidative stress and antioxidants in our cells? Ideally, we should have more data to address these questions. Results of ongoing clinical trials and further studies will be required to extend our knowledge of the impact of antioxidant supplements on health. One way to extend our knowledge about the effects of supplemental vitamins on health would be to test for benefits and harms of supplements before they come to the market. This would entail fair testing of all commercial ingested products with claimed health benefits, as we do with pharmaceutical drugs. The bigger question is, how do you test them? It's possible, and I've referred to several studies, but they cost hundreds of millions of dollars and take many years to complete. In addition, many other variables in the individual subjects are not controlled for and could be hard to control for. True, if the studies are large enough, these variables will have less of an effect, but the studies are challenging to execute, and the black-and-white readout of "disease" or "no disease" is hard to determine with current technologies.

All of these questions, and our limited answers, bring me back to the promise of emerging technologies in development that can help resolve the current confusion surrounding the vitamin debate. Proteomics allows us to get a snapshot of all of the proteins in the blood. If we took a sample from a thousand people after they had no lycopene in their diet for a certain period, then repeated that experiment with lycopene supplementation (it would probably be best to perform two subsequent studies: one with pills and another with lycopene-rich foods), and then we queried the resultant profiles versus a large cardiovascular-outcome data set, we could ask, what's the difference in cardiovascular risk between someone who is filled with lycopene and another person who's been deprived of lycopene? Correlative studies such as this could yield the pilot data for the required prospective studies. We could know more precisely who might benefit from a nutrient such as lycopene, which is prominently found in tomatoes.

I chose lycopene in the above example because it's frequently touted as a hero among anticancer nutrients, as well as the chief reason to eat tomatoes. But like so many other darlings in the nutrient world, studies haven't been able to verify the hype. The headline that Harvard published said it all: "Lycopene and Tomatoes: No Shield Against Cancer." This was in regards to a study published in September 2007, which included almost two thousand men in eight countries, that concluded carotenoids such as lycopene do not cut the odds of prostate cancer. While the researchers, many of whom were based at Oxford University in England, found that high levels of carotenoids could reduce by 60 percent the risk of an existing tumor's progressing to advanced-stage prostate cancer, they noted that carotenoids had no effect on the rate of early onset of the disease. Moreover, when FDA researchers examined eighty-one studies on lycopene, it concluded that none offered any credible evidence to support a relationship between consumption and the risk of prostate cancer. They also reviewed thirty-nine studies on tomato consumption and found limited evidence to support the notion that tomatoes and tomato-based products can trim risk.

This isn't to say that there's no value in cooking a tomato-based marinara dish tonight with chicken or pasta. Such a delicious meal might have other benefits for us, the likes of which have nothing to do with lycopene. So go ahead and enjoy a healthy meal without holding too tightly to the belief that it contains any cancer-zapping magic bullets.

Striking the Balance

Even though supplements have not proven beneficial in avoiding heart problems, foods that are sources of antioxidants are still recommended by health practitioners, myself included. Getting vitamins in food has benefits that don't necessarily occur when they are taken as supplement. For one, phytochemicals, which are naturally occurring compounds in plants that may have disease-fighting properties that can protect our health, are best delivered to the body through real foods. I don't think we may ever find a study that proves you can overdose on whole fruits and vegetables to the point you absorb a toxic or unhealthy level of certain nutrients.

Other questions are worth asking. Do we ever really know what's in our vitamins, how they are created, and whether they say what they actually are? For example, vitamin E exists in eight different forms in nature, four tocopherols and four tocotrienols. The ratio and amounts in foods are very different from those found in most pills. Just a quarter cup of sunflower seeds contains 90.5 percent of the daily value for vitamin E, yet people who take vitamin E supplements tend to consume much more than that. You only need about 22.4 IU a day, but most vitamin-E-only supplements provide more than 100 IU of the nutrient.

The vitamin and supplement industry is largely unregulated, and many trusted brands have come under fire in recent years for miserably failing quality control. Supplement and natural-food sources are not the same; the naturally occurring folate in your spinach is not the same as the synthetic folic acid in your vitamin pill. Similarly, you'll find names of chemicals and substances on supplement bottles and won't have a clue as to what they are, not to mention why you need them. When you see boron, nickel, vanadium, and manganese listed on a vitamin supplements label, for example, do you ever ask yourself if consuming these extra amounts artificially is really necessary?

We tend to assume that what a label tells us actually delivers on its promise, and that said promises are meaningful. But I implore you to question whether vitamin supplements can ever live up to Mother Nature's creations. Do we know, for instance, how to extract the good oils from a fish? Consider that to get the same amount of fish oil you would from a single serving of salmon—which is in the ballpark of three to four ounces—you would have to consume the equivalent of twenty to thirty fish-oil capsules. You should also note that not only is salmon an excellent source of omega-3 fatty acids, the good fats that inspire people to take fish-oil capsules to begin with, but it's also a great, natural source of vitamin D, selenium, protein, niacin, vitamin B12, phosphorous, magnesium, and vitamin B6. I'd rather that you obtain your nutrition from natural foods that pack a multidimensional punch than from supplements or pills that you just cannot ensure pass the QA test or even contain anything beneficial for your body.

The vitamin craze today is particularly troubling to me given how relatively easy it is to eat well in America. I'm not referring to fancy dinners at restaurants or buying your groceries at markets that charge an arm and a leg. Plenty of books can tell you how to eat "healthily," and besides, I know that you don't really need me to drive this point home. It's common knowledge now that an apple is better than an apple fritter, and that daily trips to the drive-through for your fast-food fix may not fix your cluttered arteries and high blood pressure. There's something to be said for moderation. Have a little of everything. In the spirit of bestselling author Michael Pollan's mantra: eat real (i.e., as close to nature as possible) foods. Not too much. Mostly plants. Avoid the impostors that come in packages, bottles, and boxes and have ingredients that you cannot pronounce or define without a graduate-level textbook in chemistry. I highly recommend Pollan's book *In Defense of Food* for more details.

Yet I hesitate to assume too much here because we do live in a world where obesity is taking control of too many lives. I never underestimate the intelligence and common sense of my patients, but I'm not always convinced that all of us know how to eat well, or how to keep track of how much we are really moving, as in that activity called exercise. Consider the following: *Consumer Reports* released a survey in early 2011 that reported that just one out of ten Americans admits his or her diet is unhealthy. Here's the real shocker: while four in ten admitted being "somewhat overweight," a mere 11 percent said they were very overweight or obese—a direct contradiction of previous weight measurements taken by researchers at the Centers for Disease Control and Prevention, which showed that 68 percent of Americans are overweight or obese.

I don't think this is a measure of our dishonesty, but rather another sign of our alienation and confusion when it comes to food. Often, the giant disconnect originates from how foods are marketed to us. Many people think they are eating "healthily" when they buy diet frozen dinners, fat-free ice cream or frozen yogurt, 100 percent natural fruit juice, low-fat cheese, energy bars, diet soda, blue-corn, organic, baked tortilla chips, hundred-calorie snack packs, and so on. But if you look at the nutritional content of these foods, and the order in which the ingredients are listed, which reflects their prevalence, you're likely to find more sugar, saturated fat, salt, and ingredients with weird names than anything else. It's quite telling that the survey also found that the most commonly eaten vegetable was lettuce or salad greens; 78 percent of respondents said they eat a serving a week. But what does this typically mean? Too often it means we're eating iceberg lettuce, which has nil nutritional value, and pouring on top of it a heavy dose of salad dressing that is equally anemic in healthy nutrients despite its calorie load.

So, yes, with the help of persuasive advertisements and the addictive properties of sugar and other manufactured chemicals, we can deceive ourselves easily every day in our choices. A balanced diet should naturally allow you to strike the right balance of nutrients to support a healthy state. The proverbs "Diet cures more than doctors" and "An apple a day keeps the doctor away," which some have translated to "Food is medicine," can be hard truths to swallow, quite literally. Sure, it'd be nice to know that we can pop a pill and fill in all the gaps in our nutrition, but the science just doesn't support this. Even when we're not eating the healthiest diet, there's no proof that a multivitamin or nutrient-packed pill or capsule is the right tool to seal up any dietary holes. We would do much better to exert our efforts in trying to eat better, and learning how to do so, and our money would be much better spent on quality ingredients than it would on expensive supplements. We need to read labels. We need to be honest with ourselves in our kitchens.

I'd also like to add here that I'm not the only one who has stopped taking a multivitamin and committed to paying more attention to what I put into my mouth. I'm happy to report that I've got a few fellow colleagues in my camp who now save themselves hundreds of dollars a year. David Katz, M.D., MPH, director of the Prevention Research Center at Yale University School of Medicine, no longer recommends multivitamins to most of his patients, nor does he take them himself, and Kathleen Fairfield, M.D., associate chief of medicine at Maine Medical Center and coauthor of the 2002 *JAMA* article that recommended multivitamins as a prudent health measure, has also ceased taking her daily dose. The added bonus to ditching your vitamins is that you'll automatically think seriously about your nutritional habits and be more ambitious with your grocery shopping. Soon you'll begin to do your grocery shopping with resolve, hoping to find the best, most nutrient-packed ingredients to create your next family meal. Beware, however, as looks can be deceiving at the market—especially in the "fresh" produce section.

Don't Ask for Asparagus Unless . . .

Most of us enter the grocery store with an idea of what we want to buy. We may even bring a list. The American diet has evolved to cater to our daily cravings. Many of us can't entertain the idea of shopping on a whim because that would take too long and be an exasperating exercise in indecision. But what if you asked one simple question: what fruits and vegetables just came in today? If it's asparagus, then you're in luck if that's what you had hoped for.

The answer to that single query can result in your getting the biggest bang for your caloric buck in the produce section. You'll get your hands on the most nutrient-dense fruits and vegetables available to you. Of course you could do even better by visiting your local farmers' market for the latest pickings, but if you find yourself in a typical chain supermarket, this question can be instructive and time-saving. If nothing looks good and if nothing came in recently, then head on over to the frozen section and opt for a package of fresh frozen. Yes, it's better than the stuff that's been sitting out for days, after no less than a day or so traveling in a truck to reach the supermarket. "Fresh produce" is actually not as fresh as we'd like to believe or are *led* to believe.

This is not a trivial point. When fruits fall from a tree, they immediately begin to degrade. Nature intended for this to happen so that the fruits' nutrients could be incorporated back into the soil to nourish the tree and produce another generation of juicy, nutritious fruit. The same is true for vegetables; once they are harvested, their internal chemistry begins to change. The fruits and vegetables turn on the genes (which had been dormant) to self-degrade soon after they have been picked. By the time the vast majority of produce reaches the bins and aisles of your local supermarket, it doesn't contain nearly the same volume of nutrients as when picked. If fruits and vegetables are picked before they are ripe, which many of them are to help them endure the long shipment, this gives them less time to develop a full spectrum of vitamins and minerals. Outward signs of ripening may still occur, but these vegetables will never have the same nutritive value as if they had been allowed to fully ripen on the vine. In addition, during the long haul from farm to fork, fresh fruits and vegetables are exposed to lots of heat and light, which also degrade some nutrients, especially delicate vitamins such as C and the B vitamin thiamin. What we end up with in our mouths is a nutrient-poor product that may also contain some degradative products that we would like to avoid. The enzymes involved can be halted by cold temperatures, hence the recommendation to use frozen foods as a fail-safe.

Fruits and vegetables chosen for freezing tend to be processed at their peak ripeness, a time when—as a general rule—they are most nutrient-packed. Freezing and packaging produce require techniques that lock in freshness and nutrients. Although the first step of freezing vegetables—blanching them in hot water or steam to kill bacteria and arrest the action of food-degrading enzymes—causes some water-soluble nutrients such as vitamin C and the B vitamins to break down or leach out, the subsequent flash-freeze locks the vegetables in a relatively nutrient-rich state.

> Wine growers are exceptionally aware of their grapes' fragility once they have been plucked from their stems. Top-tier vintners will only create wine using grapes that have spent little time—sometimes just minutes—going from vineyard to winery where the processing commences. The difference in taste is tremendous. It doesn't surprise me that mass-produced wines share similar flavors and that their chemistry can often leave you feeling lousier the next day than had you consumed a well-crafted bottle.

When vegetables are in season, buy them fresh and ripe when they are "just in" or can be bought at a farmers' market. But remember that "off-season," frozen vegetables will also give you a high concentration of nutrients. Go for many colors, as nature segregates nutrients by color; the blend of nutrients that make a carrot orange are different, but equally health-supporting, from those that make spinach green. To maximize the number of varying nutrients you consume, you're better off eating a yellow bell pepper and a red one than two of any single color. And please don't insult the produce by letting it sit in your kitchen's fruit bowl or "crisper" in the refrigerator. Eat fruits and vegetables soon after purchase, including the frozen variety. Over many months, even the nutrients in frozen vegetables inevitably degrade. It helps to steam or microwave rather than boil your produce to minimize the loss of water-soluble vitamins.

For a comprehensive list of nutritious fish to buy, check out the Monterey Bay Aquarium Seafood Watch website at www.seafoodwatch.org. Their list will help you determine which types of fish to buy based on where it's caught, how it's caught, and whether it contains high levels of toxins. Some seafood is better to eat from farmed varieties, whereas others are best eaten when they are wild-caught. For additional information about the mercury content of fish, you can also check the US FDA's website http://www.fda.gov/food/foodsafety/product-specificinformation/seafood/foodbornepathogenscontaminants/methylmercury/ucm115644.htm.

As many of us already know, another important source of nutrition—and a natural source of vitamin D—is fish. Here are some general guidelines about how to find the best seafood. If you live within a hundred miles of an ocean coast or a clean source of fresh fish such as some of the Great Lakes, by all means seek out fresh fish when it's available, which means it is local and in season. But if you aren't near a coast, or even if you are and would like something out of season, don't disregard frozen fish. Modern freezing techniques make many of the fish in the freezer section superior to those on the shelf nearby. Why? Because lots of fish are now frozen on the boat, just minutes after being caught, with flash-freezing units that maintain a temperature far below the typical home freezer. Many "fresh" fish are in fact previously frozen, and while most reputable fishmongers will state this on the card identifying the fish, not all do.

Junk the Juicer

As I was writing this book, I learned that one of the biggest trends in the United States in 2011 was juicing. Not that this fad hadn't already taken hold in many health and wellness circles throughout the country. Apparently, we like to juice. Juice bars have been cropping up in health-conscious towns, in gyms, and even at swanky restaurants, where it's become part of the foodie scene. If you flip on the television some Saturday morning, you'll likely find a new type of juicer on the market guaranteed to change the way you think about getting your fruits and vegetables. Some are marketed to boost your immune system, stir your metabolism, and make you a happier person.

Here's what I ask myself when I peer into the rich colors of a juicy blend: Does the body really like consuming ten carrots all at once? Or a whole head of broccoli? I know that if I were to eat these things whole, I wouldn't consume that much and that I might feel a bit sick if I tried. But the more important question to ask is whether the original nutrients in the fruits and vegetables, which now comprised in a tall glass of juice, are in fact the same. I think not.

Oxygen, as we've seen, is a powerful oxidant. It changes the chemistry of molecules in an instant when it steals electrons. As soon as we expose the inner flesh of a fruit or vegetable to the oxygen-rich air, guess what? We oxidize it on the spot, in fractions of a second—especially if we subject the fruit or vegetable to the disruptive power of a blender. We change its whole makeup and the nutrition that went with it. There's a reason why Tropicana sells most of its juices in opaque, nontransparent containers that are refrigerated. They've been in the business a long time. They know how to preserve the nutrients in their product as much as possible. Other companies, not so much. I won't name anyone other than to say watch out for juice blends sold in clear glass or plastic, which makes them sensitive to light. By the time they reach our interiors, their interiors could be worthless. As I write this, Tropicana is shifting over to clear glass containers for some of its products to compete better in the marketplace given the array of attractive see-through containers from other brands that are gaining ground. All I'll say is that it's a shame that marketing trumps health. While the peddlers of juice drinks like to refer to all the studies about the benefits of consuming more fresh fruits and vegetables, they fail to mention that these studies don't have anything to do with juice products. They are taken from studies done on whole foods. That's like comparing, excuse the joke, apples to oranges.

When foods break down, they degrade into chemicals that we don't yet understand the effects of. Vitamin C, for instance, which is an unstable molecule in the presence of oxygen, degrades pretty quickly, and one of its degradatory products, diketogulonic acid, has never been fully studied in humans. Vitamin A in food is also unstable, so it's often administered in vitamins in the form of compounds called all-trans-retinyl acetate or all-trans-retinyl palmitate. There is significant degradation of even these more stable compounds, into multiple derivatives. The ratio of these derivatives depends on the amount of light, heat, fat, and oxygen present and is, in general, unpredictable. Such degradation is especially true with vitamin A–fortified foods such as cereals. The label may indicate the activity when the product was made ("10 percent daily value of vitamin A palmitate"), but many times this has no correlation with what is in the food when we eat it. Some studies have shown that more than 90 percent of the all-trans-retinyl palmitate used to fortify cereal is gone after six to eight weeks at room temperature. Do these degradatory products have unknown side effects? This is, of course, something for us consumers and foodies to think about—and for researchers to study further.

Right about now, I hope that you're not in a semi-panic and thinking about what this means for other kitchen staples such as food processors, blenders, and, for millions of health-conscious new parents, "organic" pureed baby food. Remember what I said in the beginning of this book: a lot of my musings are merely exercises in thought. Whole foods will always be better than processed, and I think we can all agree on that. Until babies can eat solid foods, they get plenty of what they need from breast milk, formula, and, yes, even mushy baby foods probably created in a pulverizer.

Mining and Minding the Microbiome

Before we move on, I need to mention one more fact for your consideration. We are all different in how we metabolize our food, absorb its nutrients, and need or use the nutrients. This area of nutrition has to be personalized and will be in the future when new technologies become available that will allow each of us to tune in to our personal nutritional needs. Certainly genetics will play a role here, too, but the larger role will be played by the microbiome—the bacteria that fill your intestinal tract and that participate in your digestion, metabolism, and overall health.

We each have bacteria in our GI tract. Within the body of a healthy adult, microbial cells are estimated to outnumber human cells by a factor of ten to one. Each person shelters about 100 trillion microbes; by comparison, the human body is made up of only around 10 trillion cells. These microbial cells (bacteria, fungi, and viruses), however, remain largely unstudied, leaving their influence upon human development, physiology, immunity, and nutrition almost entirely unknown. Recently, the NIH launched the Human Microbiome Project (HMP; you can learn more at www.hmpdacc

.org) with the mission of generating resources enabling comprehensive characterization of the human microbiota and analysis of its role in human health and disease.

In fact, the differences in the GI flora are a viable explanation for the differences in some cancer rates between China and the United States. Take, for example, the risk of prostate cancer. For men in the United States, the risk of developing prostate cancer is about 17 percent. For men who live in rural China, however, it's a scant 2 percent. But when Chinese men move to the Western culture, their risk increases substantially after a decade.

We had assumed this was due to diet—after all, so much can be blamed on the Western diet, and certainly immigrants probably start devouring our processed, packaged foods like the rest of us when they land in the United States—but it turns out that the microbiome plays a major role here. It controls how you metabolize your food, how fast and how much you absorb, and what enters your bloodstream, thereby affecting your hormone levels among other things. In turn, this influences the risk of developing certain cancers, such as prostate or breast.

It's common to categorize people by blood type, or in some cases by ethnicity. In the future, we'll also begin to type people by "bug"— by the prevailing bacteria that inhabit their digestive tracts. In one of the more provocative studies to emerge, published in April 2011 in the journal *Nature*, a team of researchers led by Peer Bork of the European Molecular Biology Laboratory in Heidelberg, Germany, reported on three distinguishable "types" of people based on their microbiome. Each of the three types is composed of a different balance of species. People with type 1, for example, have high levels of bacteria called *Bacteroides*. In type 2, on the other hand, *Bacteroides* is relatively rare, while the genus *Prevotella* is unusually common. Part of Bork's discovery of these types of people came out of finding no link between what they call enterotypes, which are the different balances of species in a microbiome, and the ethnic background of the European, American, and Japanese subjects they studied. In other words, two Americans don't necessarily harbor the same type of bacterial ecosystem just as they may not share the same blood type. But the characteristics of their individual bacterial ecosystems could define each of their risk factors for certain diseases. Bork's team also couldn't find a connection between microbiome types and sex, weight, health, or age. They are now trying to figure out why, thinking that one possibility is that we are each randomly colonized by different pioneering species of gut microbes as infants. The microbes alter the gut so that only certain species can follow them.

Whatever the cause of the different enterotypes, they may end up having discrete effects on people's health. Gut microbes aid in food digestion and synthesize vitamins, using enzymes our own cells cannot make. Bork and his colleagues have found that each of the types makes a unique balance of these enzymes. Enterotype 1 produces more enzymes for making vitamin B7 (also known as biotin), for example, and enterotype 2 more enzymes for vitamin B1 (thiamine). I doubt that there are only a handful of enterotypes, and that in the future we'll come to know dozens if not hundreds of uniquely different clusters of enterotypes that can help inform personalized health strategies across a broad spectrum. Imagine a day when you can know how to tweak your diet in ways attuned to your personal enterotype, allowing you to effortlessly and permanently lose weight, gain sustainable energy, successfully manage and treat a chronic illness, or even end an intestinal disorder that has been the bane of your existence for as long as you can remember.

The discovery of the blood types A, B, AB, and O had a major effect on how doctors practice medicine. They could limit the chances that a patient's body would reject a blood transfusion by making sure the donated blood was of a matching type. The discovery of enterotypes could someday lead to medical applications of its own, and they will go beyond just helping people customize their diets. Drug prescriptions will also likely be tailored to match people's enterotypes, which has the potential to revolutionize an industry that's currently overly reliant on blind trial and error. Later in this book, when I cover the study of proteins and its applicability to the pharmaceutical industry, we'll see how an understanding of the body's bacterial ecosystem can help us "listen to" the dynamic conversation that's taking place between our cells. Bacteria obviously have their own DNA operating within us, and newly emerging technologies are finally helping us tune into these bacteria and their effects on us, for better or worse.

One overarching feature that studies on the microbiome are revealing is the diversity of bacteria in the human body, akin to a rain forest. Different regions of the body are home to different combinations of species. From one person to another, we're finding tremendous variety. I could have an entirely different colony of bacteria thriving in my mouth than you, which affects whether my diet helps me to maintain a healthy digestive system. In the future, perhaps I'll know more about my unique enterotype to keep my digestive system running as smoothly as possible.

Within the next ten years researchers will uncover mysteries of the microbiome and begin to find ways in which we can manipulate it to support health. The microbiome—not levels of vitamin D, for example—may explain why people who live at higher latitudes have a higher risk of developing cancer. People who live at different latitudes have different types of bacteria growing within them. I could easily envision that if you have a high risk for breast cancer based on your personal genome, doctors may adjust your microbiome in such a way as to mitigate some of the risk. Thus the combination of technologies will win here.

In addition to the active interaction that takes place every minute of the day between your digestive tract and microbiome, another big player on this field that many of us forget about is the brain. It lends a powerful voice to the conversation going on between your gut and "feelings."

A Gut Feeling

The importance of having a healthy digestive tract cannot be understated. As humans, we perceive feelings from our bodily functions, our state of well-being, our energy and stress levels, and our mood and disposition. How do we have these feelings? Understanding the neural processes that go on in the body that tell us how we feel is an area of intense study. One of the ways in which our bodies relay signals of health in their intricate networks of hormones and neurotransmitters is by creating special connections between the various systems of our physiology.

A growing body of research in recent years, thanks to breakthroughs in neuroscience and people like Emeran Mayer at UCLA's School of Medicine, has demonstrated an intimate, two-way connection between the brain and the digestive system. It is quite remarkable—so stunningly complex is this relationship that the gut can be considered the largest sensory organ in the body. Michael Gershon, an expert in the nascent field of neurogastroenterology and author of the 1998 book *The Second Brain*, calls our gut just that: it's our second brain, with powers that go far beyond making sure that things keep moving through and out of our colon. Here's the gist of it: First, the gut sends information to the brain via the vagus nerve and so-called spinal afferent nerves. The purpose of this gut-to-brain signaling is to provide input to a hierarchy of reflex loops at different levels of the central nervous system, including the spinal cord, brain stem, hypothalamus, and a special area of the brain called the primary interoceptive cortex. Through this signaling, the brain receives information about what's going on in the gut. Likewise, the central nervous system sends information back to the gut to ensure optimal functioning during sleep, fasting, and digestion. After all, without all this communication back and forth, it would be impossible to control our eating behavior and digestion.

What's truly amazing is that the gut actually has its own little network that allows it to respond to the brain and signal when something isn't right. This process ensures that what the gut does is always well coordinated with your overall state. In addition to nerve signals, the gut also emits hormonal signals that reach the brain directly or through stimulation of the sensory nerves. For example, certain gut hormones can transmit sensations of fullness and hunger. Similarly, when there's inflammation going on somewhere in the intestine, the gut can also trigger brain functions such as pain, fatigue, increased sleep, and a feeling of "being sick." In other words, if you suffer from a disease, illness, or infection that affects your gut, so much of how you feel will be attributed to your gut's influences on your brain, and can even have an impact on how you think, how much pain you experience, how well you sleep, and what your energy levels are.

Because the gut sends an enormous amount of information to an area of the brain responsible for our feelings of self-awareness and well-being, the health of our gut can be a much bigger factor in our perception of health than we might imagine. For example, the uneasy feeling—that knot or swarm of butterflies—in our bellies that some of us experience when we're worried, anxious, scared, or angry are all sensations that may get stored in a unique type of memory, called a "body map," and which can influence our later decisions in similar situations.

It should come as no surprise that improving the relationship between our brain and our gut can improve our overall health and sense of wellness. Researchers of this brain-gut connection point out that eating a healthy diet that is low in fat and refined sugars, high in natural fibers, low in calories, and taken in several small portions during the day should help promote the natural balance our body wants to maintain. Conversely, an oversize, high-fat, high-calorie meal, particularly when eaten late at night when our digestion is supposed to go into its fasting mode, is likely to cause intestinal disturbances and associated feelings of distress.

Can we *think* our way to a healthier gut? This part of the research is still in its infancy, but the findings thus far are fascinating. By becoming more aware of pleasant gut sensations and learning to think about occasional negative sensations such as fullness, abdominal pain, and discomfort as normal rather than serious, you may, over time, avoid feeling that discomfort. This may all sound abstract and difficult to understand, but suffice it to say that the brain-gut connection is real and more bewildering than we ever thought possible. This knowledge tells us that achieving the healthiest gut you can through your diet and lifestyle choices is paramount. It plays into our emotions, sense of well-being, and *feelings* more than you know or have ever appreciated.

Not surprisingly, this latest research has also shed more light on how gut bacteria influence our health, and how adding certain probiotics to support the good bacteria in our gut may positively influence the responsiveness of our body's stress system, particularly with regard to pain sensitivity, gut inflammation, and the regulation of our emotions. Researchers are currently looking at the possible role that some strains of intestinal bacteria have in obesity, inflammatory and functional GI disorders, chronic pain, autism, and depression. They are also examining the role that these bacteria play in our emotions. Perhaps we'll find one day that a certain strain of bacteria in the gut can predict whether someone is generally happy and optimistic, or foul-natured and pessimistic.

Understanding the gut connection to our overall health can help us to appreciate more the choices we make and what pressures we encounter throughout any given day. Such pressures don't necessarily have to be psychological or stress-related. Some of the most pervasive pressures that we endure daily, which can have sneaky, unintended consequences to our long-term health, arise from right under our feet. Literally.

le

t your nutrition—including naturally occurring vitamins and minerals—from real, whole food that is as close to nature as possible. Don't trust anything that comes out of a blender, juicer, or glass jar. Buy frozen fruits and vegetables or "fresh flash-frozen" over what many supermarkets sell as just fresh. It's hard to summarize nutritional recommendations in a list, but below is a list of general recommendations. Understanding the complex nature of nutrition is a more important principle, but lists can be helpful tools:

1. Moderation.
2. Eat on a regular schedule—it doesn't matter how many meals, just regular timing. No snacking. (You'll learn the importance of maintaining such strict regularity shortly.)
3. Eat cold-water fish a minimum of three times per week (e.g., salmon, sardines, tuna, rainbow trout, anchovies, herring, halibut, cod, black cod, mahimahi, etc.). Exception: It's better to avoid fish than to consume any fish that is not recommended by SeafoodWatch.org, which keeps a running record of safe, ocean-friendly seafood.
4. Choose a multicolored diet.
5. Drink red wine (one a glass a night) five nights per week—unless you're at high risk for breast cancer.
6. Eat a good-fat diet—not a low-fat diet.
7. Read Michael Pollan's *In Defense of Food*—it's the best book on food.

9

Hot and Heavy

What NFL Football Players and Nuns Can Teach Us about Deadly Inflammation—and How to Control It

When I tell my patients and friends to wear good, comfortable shoes, my advice is as simple and straightforward as it sounds. Can the shoes we wear affect whether we collapse of a heart attack ten years sooner than had we just kept with cozy sneakers our whole life? After you read the information in this chapter, I'll let you be the judge. It all starts with a discussion about inflammation.

The concept of inflammation has been tossed around a lot in recent years. As with vitamin D, it seems to have its own publicist because the word crops up in numerous health-related articles today—both as *inflammation* and its antidote, *anti-inflammatory*. I'll assume that you have a vague notion of what it's about given casual exposure to the topic in such articles and the definition I offered briefly earlier in the book, but I'll also presume that you'd like to know a little more.

We're all familiar with the kind of inflammation that accompanies cuts and bruises on our skin—the pain, swelling, and redness that emerges. Or the ache of a torn muscle, broken bone, and sting of a sunburn. If you suffer from allergies or arthritis, you're also tuned in to what some types of inflammation can feel like in other ways—sneezing, itching, rashes, hives, joint soreness and gnawing pain, etc. But inflammation goes much deeper than that and can happen in your organs and systems without your even feeling or knowing it.

Although inflammation is part of our bodies' natural defense mechanism against foreign invaders such as bad bacteria, viruses, and toxins, too much inflammation can be harmful. When inflammation runs rampant or goes awry, it can disrupt the immune system and lead to chronic problems and/or disease. It's like turning up the furnace to keep us warm and comfortable. If that furnace doesn't turn off once a certain temperature is reached, then our environment is going to get hot, uncomfortable, and dangerous. Soon enough, things in that environment will start to become adversely affected.

Inflammation may not seem related to many conditions and afflictions, but volumes of international research prove just how insidious chronic inflammation can be on the body. Certain kinds of inflammation have been linked to our most troubling degenerative diseases today, including heart disease, Alzheimer's disease, cancer, autoimmune diseases, diabetes, and accelerated aging. I can't think of a chronic condition that hasn't been associated with inflammation, which results in an imbalance in our system that stimulates negative effects on our health, just as many of the other inputs we've discussed—including excess vitamins, antioxidants, calories, etc.

At the center of inflammation is the concept of oxidative stress, which, in a rudimentary sense, is like a biological type of "rusting" of our organs and tissues. This can happen both on the outside, causing wrinkles and premature aging, and on the inside, where it can stiffen our blood vessels, damage cell membranes, and essentially wreak havoc on our precious interior designs. Obviously, the human body doesn't rust like metal left out in the rain and sun, but the rusting analogy helps to understand the chemical reactions that take place during oxidative stress. I mentioned before that oxidation is a normal part of everyday living, but oxidation in overdrive can become a problem. New technologies will allow us to further understand this process of inflammation and how we can gain control of it for the better. The goal will be to develop metrics for quantifying inflammation and segregating various types of inflammation, from good to bad. Some inflammation we want, and some we don't. The JUPITER study I chronicled in chapter 2 was among the first to really identify inflammation as the undercurrent to illness. The buildup of inflammation—not necessarily cholesterol—is what can lead to a heart attack. The actual sequence of actions that takes place beginning with inflammation and ending in an actual heart attack is complex, involving changes to the coronary artery and blood vessels that nourish the heart, but the outcome is the same: an increased risk for a life-threatening cardiovascular event.

When Your Job Is Hazardous to Your Health

Once you understand that blocking unnecessary inflammation as much as you can is key, the next question becomes how—how do you know where and why it's happening and attempt to control it? This is not always the easiest question to answer, but what you might not think about is the chronic inflammation you could be exposing yourself to in daily living that can be controlled. I wonder, for example, when a woman wears uncomfortable heels, what is that constant, low-grade irritation doing to her overall system? It's no surprise that certain jobs bear risks, and that being a tree feller, crab fisherman, or football player means that you sit somewhere higher on the mortality charts. These are extreme examples of professions in which one is more likely to die prematurely than to wither away slowly far into old age than the people who opted for less risky jobs. I'm not about to equate a corporate executive who wears uncomfortable shoes with a crab fisherman braving high seas and blistering conditions, but the question remains: how much does inflammation play into the general mortality tables across the spectrum of circumstances, and how much pressure causes a damaging result? Let's take one extreme and consider a football player who gets a lot of playtime and, as a consequence, takes or makes a lot of hits. We actually have statistics here to consider, published in 2006 as part of a study,* and they are quite sobering:

- Heavy (overweight) NFL players are twice as likely to die before the age of fifty.
- Twenty-eight percent of all pro football players born in the last century who qualified as obese died before their fiftieth birthday, compared with 13 percent who were less overweight.
- One of every sixty-nine players born since 1955 is now dead. Twenty-two percent of those players died of heart diseases; 19 percent died from homicides or suicides.
- Seventy-seven percent of those who died of heart diseases qualified as obese, even during their playing days, and they were two and a half times more likely to die of coronaries than their trimmer teammates.
- Only 10 percent of deceased players born from 1905 through 1914 were obese while active. Today, more

---

*The study came from a Scripps Howard News Service analysis of 3,850 professional football players who have died in the last century. More specifically, the Scripps Howard study created a computer database of the deaths of 3,850 former professional football players using records assembled by professional football statistician David Neft and his colleagues.

than half of all players on NFL rosters are categorized as obese.

- The average weight in the NFL has grown by 10 percent since 1985 to a current average of 248 pounds. The heaviest position, offensive tackle, went from 281 pounds two decades ago to 318 pounds.

Without a doubt, we can point fingers at excess weight and, as a result, premature heart disease as a potent killer among football players. Body size is well documented to be inversely related to longevity, as both tallness and heaviness have been linked to increased early-life mortality in epidemiological studies. It makes sense that football linemen maintaining a high body mass for competitive reasons would likely be sacrificing years of life for their large size. Although it would seem logical to say that a football player's high level of exercise could protect him from cardiovascular risks associated with large size, this just doesn't prove to be the case. The pros of physical activity cannot cancel or supersede the cons of excess weight. Several studies have confirmed this, for large athletes are not in peak physical condition—their time spent exercising heavily does not outweigh the negative health effects of their large size. This research has shot down the concept that you can be both fat and fit. Excess weight is thought to be so damaging because of the hidden march of inflammation behind the scenes.

Whether we're considering the detrimental effects of excessive body weight or routine hits from other players, the common denominator here is inflammation. In all of the symptoms that football players exhibit as a consequence of their profession, the one that surely keeps on going is inflammation, which for many of them sets in motion a sequence of biological events that can lead to a heart attack. Long after a football player has hung up his helmet, his body is trying to heal itself, and that pathway back to health likely entails some inflammation, which you'll recall is part of the natural healing process. As this book was going to press, the news hit that NFL Hall of Famer Lee Roy Selmon died two days after being hospitalized for a stroke. He was fifty-six. Though he was far from the image of an obese man who looked dangerously close to having a sudden cardiac event, the inflammation he'd endured years ago on the field had other consequences for him. Would he have died had he not been a football player? We'll never know, but the facts of his profession's history share a similar, grim theme.

In addition to the increased risk for heart attack and stroke among those who suffer chronic inflammation, people can also up their risk for cancer as a result of that untamed inflammation. In areas where a football player, for instance, has sustained repeated blows, such as the head, shoulders, trunk, etc., DNA in that region could have been irreparably damaged. It's interesting to note that some individuals who've been diagnosed with cancer in particular locations of their bodies can link that specific area to a previous trauma or injury—football player or not. When Bruce Feiler, a popular writer on faith and author of *The Council of Dads*, told his triumphant cancer survival story at TEDMED in 2010, he shared how when he learned of his seven-inch bone tumor in his left femur in 2008 at the age of forty-four, he couldn't help but cast his mind back to the day he experienced a terrible accident on his bicycle as a young boy that had damaged that same leg. Coincidence? Probably not.

Inflammation's Path of Destruction

DNA is incredibly resilient. We all have lots of built-in mechanisms to send in troops to repair DNA when it's broken. And it's not just one mechanism. As I've already discussed, the human body is wonderfully redundant in a lot of ways. We have backup plans at virtually every corner and in every critical reaction. How else could we survive all that we do in life? Indeed, the human body is fail-safe . . . up to a certain threshold. None of us knows where that threshold resides within us, though. That's the million-dollar question that will never be answered. In the face of chronic inflammation, such as the case with repeated trauma or a prolonged injury or illness, the body can shut down DNA repair. It does this to conserve energy; it goes into survival mode. DNA repair is an incredibly energy-intensive, arguably the most labor-intensive chore that the body performs. When the body is shouldering the weight of chronic inflammation, it must shunt the energy it takes to deal with DNA repair to the demanding inflammation.

When the body's DNA repair shop is closed, the body can become vulnerable to cancer and other diseases. Although this is just a hypothesis, it's intriguing and is presently being tested. Think about it: when inflammation subsides, normalcy ensues, and the DNA repair shop reopens for business, but it could be too late. Cancerous cells could already have started to propagate, at which point the inherent DNA repair system is no longer effective. It cannot fix the cancer.

The clear association between inflammation and cancer is real and has many examples. One of the most exciting recent studies was published in the June 22, 2010, issue of the *Journal of the American College of Cardiology*. The analysis of two dozen randomized, controlled trials that were studying therapies for cholesterol found that each 10 mg/dl higher increment of HDL cholesterol (the good cholesterol) was associated with a relative 36 percent *lower* risk of cancer. The relationship persisted even after adjusting for LDL cholesterol (the bad cholesterol), age, body mass index (BMI), diabetes, sex, and smoking status. The researchers were quick to note that these association studies cannot prove cause and effect, although it's been suggested that HDL may have anti-inflammatory and antioxidant properties that could potentially fight cancer.

Other types of inflammation, such as repeated head trauma, clearly can do more than inflict minuscule, albeit long-term, damage to DNA that opens the door for cancer to develop later in one's lifetime. On a more short-term timeline, it can mangle the brain's physical components. Movement of the brain within the skull can damage nerve cells and synapses, and a research group at Purdue University hypothesized that there may be additive effects of repeated head trauma even if individual impacts do not produce any symptoms. To test our their theory, they conducted an experiment using helmet-based sensors, video, cognitive tests, and functional MRI (fMRI) to determine neurological changes in high school football players due to head trauma.

Data from the helmet sensors reported forces of up to 100 g sustained upon impact (for reference, most roller coasters expose riders to forces of only 5 g). Players that showed symptoms (concussion) were expected to have neurological changes and indeed did. Notably, though, of the players who received a high number of or unusually hard impacts, half of those who showed no symptoms still suffered cognitive impairments, based on cognitive tests and brain scans performed before, during, and after the season. They showed deficits in their memory recall and also altered activation in a part of the brain in proximity to the most frequent area of impact. This was a significant finding; players who didn't have any symptoms likely went on playing after hard impacts, not realizing they were risking further head trauma, and more serious neurologic injury and intellectual deterioration.

Complicating this already dismal picture for aspiring football stars is the cautionary tale of Owen Thomas, a popular six-foot-two, 240-pound junior lineman for the University of Pennsylvania. In the spring of 2010, this promising young student-athlete hanged himself in his off-campus apartment after what friends and family described as a sudden and uncharacteristic emotional collapse. He had no previous history of depression. A brain autopsy revealed the same trauma-induced disease found in more than twenty deceased National Football League players: chronic traumatic encephalopathy (CTE), a disease linked to depression and impulse control primarily found in NFL players, two of whom also committed suicide in the last ten years.

The doctors who examined Thomas's brain tissue cautioned that his suicide should not be attributed solely or even primarily to the damage in his brain, given the prevalence of suicide among college students in general. But they did say that a twenty-one-year-old's having developed the disease so early raised the possibility that it played a role in his death and provided arresting new evidence that the brain damage found in NFL veterans can afflict younger players, as damage starts accruing early.

Thomas never had a diagnosis of a concussion on or off the football field or even complained of a headache, although he reportedly was the kind of player who might have ignored the symptoms to stay on the field. Because of this, his CTE—whose only known cause is repetitive brain trauma—must have developed from concussions he dismissed or from the thousands of subconcussive collisions he withstood in his dozen years of football, most of them while his brain was developing.

Thomas had everything going for him and didn't fall into that category of students who appeared doomed to become another suicide statistic. He was bright enough to be attending Penn's Wharton School, one of the best undergraduate business programs in the country. He played freshman football and then started the last two seasons on the varsity, earning second-team all–Ivy League honors in 2009 and helping lead the Quakers to the Ivy title. Popular, charismatic, and destined for success, Thomas left no note and still had his cell phone in his pocket at the time he killed himself, a potential sign that he was acting on impulse, not forethought. Lack of impulse control is a consistent manifestation of how executive function can be compromised by CTE, which is characterized by the presence of twisted proteinlike formations in the frontal lobe of the cerebral cortex that resemble the plaques found in Alzheimer's patients' brains. His brain fogged by these intrusive proteins, Thomas's ability to think rationally was compromised.

The point of this story is not so much about determining what exactly precipitated Thomas's rare condition and eventual death as it is about the fragility of the human body (and in this case, brain) when confronted with chronic inflammation. As an active football player, Thomas endured relentless inflammation that changed the chemistry in his brain. Could genes and other environmental factors such as psychological stress have been a catalyst? While we cannot discredit these other potential factors in his demise, the undercurrent of inflammation likewise cannot be ignored. At the heart of CTE is an inflammation that has the power to inflict lasting and, in some cases, catastrophic damage on a brain—even a young one.

Thank Heaven for Nuns

The brain is a beautiful microcosm of the body—an exceedingly complex organ that we barely understand. We may only use a fraction of our brain's capacity, but what's more significant is that we only understand a small fraction of how our brains work and what can trigger illness and dementia. Although it's now widely accepted in the medical community that inflammation is an underlying theme in the instigation and progression of brain disease, we still lack the data to fully comprehend what makes one person's brain falter, sometimes at an early age, while someone else's remains healthy and sharp. The dearth in research over the last century can partly be attributed to a scarcity in donated brains. When people die, brains are often left intact, rarely finding their ways into the halls of research medicine. Hopefully, though, we have a few charitable nuns and recent donors to thank in helping us understand our cerebral tissues better in the future.

One of the more intriguing studies ever to be performed on brains was the Nun Study, launched in 1986 under David Snowden of the University of Kentucky. Snowden set out to collect clues about how we can have a better quality of life as we age by following hundreds of nuns who agreed to take mental tests, fill out questionnaires, and donate their brains after they died to be examined for the telltale plaques and tangles that are the definitive diagnosis for Alzheimer's disease. A common joke among the nuns in the study became a rallying cry: "When we die, our souls will go to heaven, but our brains will go to Kentucky."

The nuns were ideal subjects for the long-term comparative study because they shared such similar life experiences, without confounding variables such as income, pregnancy, or heavy smoking and drinking. In Snowden's 2001 book, *Aging with Grace*, which chronicled his experience, he writes that one of the chief messages to be taken from the study is that upbeat attitudes and mentally active lifestyles may offer protection against the onset of implacable, and still mysterious, dementia. He also noted how the vibrancy and complexity of the prose in autobiographies of convent applicants turned out be one of the best predictors of whether they would develop Alzheimer's disease. Nuns who wrote sentences thick with ideas were less likely to develop dementia than those whose autobiographies showed a paucity of themes.

The now-famous Nun Study was just the beginning. A handful of studies are finally taking place nationwide today that use donated brains with a rich and detailed clinical history gleaned from years of memory tests and physical exams. In 2009, the National Institutes of Health awarded Rush University about $5.5 million in grants to study how epigenetic changes—chemical modifications to genes that can result from diet, aging, stress, or environmental exposure—contribute to memory formation and cognitive decline.

These studies have already unveiled surprising findings, one of which is a concept that neurologist David Bennett, director of Rush University's Alzheimer's Disease Center, calls *neural reserve*. Almost a third of the participants who died without demonstrating any marked memory loss exhibited hallmarks of Alzheimer's disease when their brains were examined by neuropathologists using high-powered microscopes. In other words, their brains contained some sort of "reserve" for functioning relatively well despite showing physical signs of disease, which are characterized by the buildup of amyloid plaques, which are found outside the neurons, and neurofibrillary tangles, which are found inside the neurons. These plaques and tangles are appropriately named; it helps to think of them as the "sticky" culprits to brain disease for their ability to clump up and "entangle" the brain's nerve cells in ways that destroy normal functioning of the brain.

The role of amyloid plaques and neurofibrillary tangles on the functioning of the brain is by no means fully understood. Most people with Alzheimer's disease show evidence of both plaques and tangles, but a small number of people with Alzheimer's only have plaques and some have only neurofibrillary tangles. But what about people who have these physical manifestations of disease but no other signs of Alzheimer's? Finding people who have both plaques and tangles but who don't show signs of Alzheimer's demonstrates how much we don't know about this disease. Bennett's explanation of neural reserve is an attempt to rectify the disparities, as he noticed patterns in those who—despite their plaques and tangles—were not diagnosed with Alzheimer's.

Neural reserve seemed to correlate largely with highly educated and socially and physically active people. Thus, according to Bennett, it may be possible to delay the onset of Alzheimer's symptoms by "building a better brain through your life experiences." Why were these people's brains so robust? Obviously, if we can figure out what these individuals were doing right, we can develop more evidence-based preventive measures to preserve our brains while we're alive and hoping to participate in life to its fullest for as long as we possibly can.

The idea that we can build better brains that defend themselves against harmful inflammation is empowering; it means we can proactively have an impact on whether our brains go to mush sooner rather than later. Alzheimer's disease is the most common form of dementia, affecting about 5.3 million Americans, and is the nation's seventh-leading cause of death. The number of cases is rising as Americans live longer from healthier lifestyles and improved health care, and it is expected to keep climbing as baby boomers reach old age. It can be devastating to watch a loved one suffer from Alzheimer's for many years. I hope that I live to see the day we can wipe this affliction off the planet and keep people's brains as robust and young as the rest of their bodies.

Not surprisingly, as this book was going to press, the game of football received another blow to its luster in the sports world when scientists at Loyola University Chicago's Stritch School of Medicine found that 35 percent of 513 retired NFL players scored poorly enough on a test for Alzheimer's symptoms to indicate dementia. Then, when the researchers looked more closely at a random sample of forty-one of those low-scoring players, they noted that the players' scores on other cognitive tests showed that their brain functions were closer to those of patients diagnosed with mild cognitive impairment (MCI) than to those of healthy people. Not everyone with MCI develops Alzheimer's disease, but the condition can be equally disheartening. If you have MCI, you'll experience memory loss, confusion, and difficulty concentrating—pretty much a milder form of the dreaded disease. Also no surprise is that these researchers surmised that NFL players have a smaller reserve of healthy brain tissue than those who haven't spent time on the field. Unfortunately, helmets don't protect the brain from this type of damage. Only staying out of the game does.

In addition to the kind of inflammation in the brain that invites physical changes such as those plaques and tangles, inflammation can take many other forms in the body as a result of illness or dysfunction, which are far more universally experienced in the general population from a young age. As you're about to find out, everyone suffers from one type of inflammation in particular at some point, which can have long-term effects that most of us don't think about.

Why Today's Annoying Flu
Can Spell Trouble Years from Now

Most of us are not football players and tree fellers. And we're probably not living like nuns, who lead pretty healthy lives by virtue of their calling's abstemious lifestyle. Because of their strict schedules and lifestyles, Roman Catholic nuns live longer than those in any other job, lasting an average of eighty-six years. We're hard at work in other settings and wearing different uniforms. But inflammation comes into our lives in a way pretty regularly that typically has nothing to do with our jobs. It strikes when we get sick. Battling a cold or flu entails a bout with inflammation as our bodies fight to rid us of the infection and return to "normal."

Much of the discomfort we feel when we catch a relentless cold or flu is from an overactive immune system. When it encounters an invader it's never before seen, which in this case is some type of virus, it tends to overreact like an irrational personality that blows everything out of proportion. This is why vaccines—the antidotes to viruses—are effective. They prepare the body's defenses to deal with a certain invader and essentially whet your immune system's appetite for the infection beforehand. So if and when the infection does strike, our immune system is already acquainted with the invader and doesn't need to respond so ferociously. Once our body has been exposed to a certain virus, it knows how to kill it quickly and keep the "memory" of that antidote in our immune system, which is why we won't suffer from the same virus twice. It's extremely rare, for example, to get the same cold twice or the exact same strain of a flu virus.

When the swine flu circled the globe in 2009, the people who were most vulnerable to the potentially fatal virus were those whose immune systems were untested or were caught off guard. This included younger generations with immune systems that had little experience fighting flus, and pregnant women whose immune systems were dampened at the time to protect the fetus. All pregnant women's immune systems tick down a notch to prevent the immune system from attacking the growing fetus as if it were an invader. Older generations had some residual protective effects from having survived other viruses that had some similarity to the swine flu but to which the younger generation hadn't been exposed. Exempt from this protection, however, were elderly individuals with other medical conditions that weakened their immunity, making these people extremely susceptible. Those who successfully battled through the flu gained the benefit of lifetime immunity, but they also endured lots of inflammation during the healing, which would include its own lasting—negative—impact.

Yet there was one exception to this negative phenomenon. Those who were already taking statins when they contracted the virus escaped exposure to excessive inflammation while their bodies got well. Statins, the drugs that block inflammation as we've seen, are one of the few drugs that will prevent you from being put on a ventilator if you come down with swine flu. For this reason, many CDC officials carry statins with them wherever they go, right alongside some meat tenderizer. Why meat tenderizer? Should an official be bitten by a feisty, potentially menacing bug, what's good for your steak is good for the bite. Meat tenderizer contains papain, which breaks down the protein toxins in the venom. A bottle of classic Adolph's is often the best treatment for jellyfish, bee, and yellow jacket stings, mosquito bites, and possibly stingray wounds. It will deactivate venom before the body absorbs and detects it and consequently sends out its soldiers in a highly reactive inflammatory process.

My hope is that we can begin to study the use of statins across a wide variety of ailments due to their lowering of inflammation. In August 2011, one headline caught my eye that confirmed this need for more studies; in layman's terms it went something like this: *"Legacy effects" of statin therapy translates to a 14 percent reduction in all kinds of deaths.* Eight years after the end of a European study that looked at the effects of taking 10 milligrams of Lipitor, researchers found the convincing evidence they needed to show that statins don't just reduce one's risk of a heart attack. They reduce one's overall risk of dying from noncardiac events, particularly respiratory illnesses and infections. Hence, taking a statin can have long-term protective effects on the body, and can even wield its positive health benefits long after the statin therapy has ended.

I suspect that we'll find new correlations like these that can help people who've never considered taking a statin. Could statins, for the sake of argument, help epileptics? All our cells' membranes have fat (lipids) in them. If I put you on Lipitor, one of the most commonly prescribed statins for lowering the risk of heart attack and stroke, I somewhat change the lipid component of your cellular membranes, and thus their electrical conductance. At the heart of epilepsy is a problem with electrical signals going back and forth in the brain's cellular communications. Do people who take statins have a lower risk of epilepsy? I don't believe this question has been answered, or even asked. We have to begin to pose questions like these in abundance across the entire spectrum of medicine using emerging technologies.

Not only does the flu come with staggering amounts of inflammation, but it leaves destructive marks in its path. No, not physical marks per se. But ghostly marks. Every time your body is exposed to prolonged, intense rounds of inflammation, such as the kind that accompanies the flu, you put a lot of wear and tear on your system as it sustains a dangerous storm of molecules. This storm, which produces a flurry of chemicals called cytokines, will age your blood vessels no matter how old or young you are at the time. Hence, you set yourself up to suffer from long-term effects of this temporary storm, however brief.

I'm a big believer in flu vaccines. If not to prevent the flu, then to at least prevent marked increases of inflammation that can come back to haunt us later in life when we grow ever more vulnerable to diseases rooted in inflammation. In 2006, the American Heart Association and the American College of Cardiology jointly recommended influenza immunization as part of comprehensive secondary prevention in persons with coronary and other atherosclerotic vascular disease.

> A mere two weeks of an inflammatory storm can harm us in ways that increase our lifetime risk of myriad illnesses, including obesity, heart attack, stroke, and cancer. Such an inflammatory storm could just be the result of recovering from a bad seasonal cold or flu.

This was based on evidence from studies that indicated that annual vaccination against seasonal influenza in people with cardiovascular conditions prevents fatal heart attacks and strokes and even reduces the risk of death from *any illness*. I firmly believe that it should also be part of primary prevention. If you choose not to get vaccinated every year, then do what you can to avoid contact with others who are sick. Practice good hygiene and stay away from people with runny noses. I don't mean to sound pedantic or unimaginative, but this kind of advice is underestimated, yet vitally important.

So with all of this in mind, let's return to the shoes. If the goal is to reduce your overall inflammation and take the load off your joints and lower back to further reduce this inflammation, then I know of no better, easier way to do this than to simply wear a good pair of shoes daily. Thankfully, lots of running-shoe companies such as Nike and Puma manufacture dress casual shoes for people such as me who want to feel comfortably cushioned all day long in formal settings. We would do well to choose a shoe that is flexible, light-weight, and well supported. Sorry, but platform pumps and stilettos don't count no matter how much you tell yourself that the shoes meet these criteria. This isn't the most difficult lifestyle change to make, and a good pair of shoes will go a long way to protect you. If you need another reason to wear athletic shoes every day, then consider how much easier it will be for you to make exercise a part of your daily life, which is another recommendation I'll make in the spirit of reducing not just inflammation, but increasing lots of other nodes in your complex system.

Health Rule

Take charge of hidden, sneaky sources of chronic inflammation that can trigger illness and disease by wearing comfortable shoes daily, getting an annual flu vaccine, and asking your doctor why you're not on a statin and baby aspirin if you're over the age of forty.

10

Running to Sit Still

The Perils of a Prolonged Perch

Everyone knows that exercise is good for us. The science is well documented and delivered through media every day with headlines reminding us that exercise fights the onset of age-related disease, cinches the waistline and makes weight control easier, promotes a sense of well-being, increases our lung capacity so we can take in more oxygen, boosts circulation to deliver nutrients to cells, reduces stress, and, yes, lowers inflammation. Moving our body has lots of anti-inflammatory action, releasing endorphins that counteract the stress hormone cortisol, among other things. That may seem counterintuitive to some of you who have experienced muscle soreness or aches and pains after a hard workout. But remember that inflammation can have positive effects in small doses; this kind of inflammation is a normal response to muscle exertion and is part of an adaptation that leads to greater stamina and strength. (After exercise it helps to ice the painful areas—don't heat them. The ice will reduce that inflammation quickly, while the heat can make matters worse, increasing your discomfort and prolonging your recovery.)

I work in a field where, for many of my patients, exercise is the last thing on their minds, but I still do what I can to get them moving. I cannot express in words how transformative it can be for those who stay as active as their bodies will let them, even those who are suffering mightily from disease. One of my all-star patients, whom I'll call Nathan, changed his life the day he was diagnosed with prostate cancer at the age of nearly eighty. This man had already led a fulfilling and successful life and had survived a near-death experience more than once. But it took the diagnosis of cancer for him to take his health seriously. He started to pay close attention to his diet and eat better, and he ditched a life of erratic schedules and created a daily routine for himself (which we'll see, in the next chapter, is critical). Part of that routine was a swim every single day. As I write this, Nathan is almost ninety years young. He continues to manage his cancer and live life to the fullest. I don't think he'd be here today if it weren't for his positive attitude and dedication to his own metrics for health.

Sickness should have little, if anything, to do with whether we exercise. If you ask people why they don't engage in regular physical activity, though, it's usually not because they are battling a serious illness. Most people lament that they just don't enjoy it. Or they don't like to sweat. Or they don't have time. Admittedly, I myself do not train for marathons or wake up in the morning thinking about a workout right away. But I do appreciate the rewards that come with regular exercise; I do find time to incorporate physical activity into my day no matter what; and I do value the scientific evidence that keeps screaming in our ears about exercise's magical effects on the body's system. When I was digging into the research to write this chapter, I was quite amazed by what I encountered in the literature. I was particularly taken aback by the history of the study of exercise because we take for granted today that we know it's good for us. I am compelled to share some of that history and evidence here in the hopes you take this advice seriously if you aren't already committed to sweating it out more than once in a while. I'll keep it short and, hopefully, sweet.

Before I do, I'll note the encouraging news that you don't have to set your sights on a competitive athletic event or even join a gym. Moving your body is easier than you think, especially when you know it's arguably the only scientifically proven "secret" to youth that doesn't require a huge investment of time or money. The bad news, however, is that you cannot just take a pill to get your exercise in. It does require some effort.

The Only Proven Fountain of Youth

It is hard to imagine a time when we didn't know that physical activity helps to keep our hearts strong and our bodies young. The Athenians, after all, invented the athlete. Legend has it that only upper-class men in Athenian society were granted athletic opportunities and trained to perfect their physical beauty through exercise; everyone else was limited to watching these men compete. But if you were living in the mid-twentieth century, and I realize that many of you were born at that time, your doctor would have expressed doubt as to the connection between physical fitness and well-being, or, more specifically, fitness and the prevention of disease. It hadn't yet been scientifically shown. As recently as the 1950s, doctors believed running would stress the heart too much. People over forty were even encouraged to move from a two-story to a one-story house to reduce their exertion.

I suppose that some people had an instinctive hunch about the benefits of exercise long before then just from their own experience and casual reflections on who lived better and longer among their family and friends. In 1873, Edward Stanley, the Earl of Derby, gave an address at Liverpool College in which he said, "Those who think they have not time for bodily exercise will sooner or later have to find time for illness." Yet, it would take more than a century after that—and more than twenty-seven hundred years since the first Olympic Games—for the fitness movement to take hold, for doctors to take exercise seriously (whether for themselves or to recommend to patients), and for people such as Jane Fonda, Joanie Greggains, and Jack LaLanne to create brands out of spreading the message about the benefits of exercise. Within just one decade doctors would go from warning their heart-attack patients to avoid exercise entirely to recommending that they resume an exercise program to help avoid future attacks.

The notion that exerting the body physically is good for health began to pique the interest of some researchers after a somewhat random large-scale study was done on bus drivers and conductors in London. In 1953, a group of British scientists led by Jeremiah Morris decided to examine the onset of heart disease in thirty-one thousand male transport workers between the ages of thirty-five and sixty-five. Morris, affectionately called Jerry by his peers, would go on to become a tireless crusader for health, and one of the world's first advocates for physical activity. But his commitment to proving the benefits of exercise happened quite haphazardly. Initially, he didn't intend to prove a connection between heart disease and level of activity per se. This would become an observation by accident, setting the course for the rest of his professional life. At the outset, Morris and his team were simply trying to "seek for relations between the kind of work men do and the incidence among them of [coronary artery disease]." Never in his wildest dreams could Morris have predicted that the data would be unleashed from this initial query and that would later transform the world to some degree.

Morris was born in Liverpool on May 6, 1910, to Jewish immigrant parents who, just a few weeks prior, had come to Britain to escape the escalating genocide in Poland. The family arrived by boat and adopted the surname of the ship's captain, and then soon settled in Glasgow, Scotland, where Morris grew up in a multilingual family and where he saw social deprivation on a daily basis. Morris began exercising as a child. His father, who was a Hebrew scholar, would take him and his brothers on four-mile walks once a week, then reward them with ice cream if they completed the walk within an hour (Morris never figured out where his father got the four miles an hour from). After returning from military service in World War II, he, along with other scientists and public health officials, became aware of the modern epidemic of coronary heart disease. The cause was unclear, but some evidence led Morris and others to suspect that occupation might be a factor. He picked an easy group of people to study, abundant in London's transportation system: double-decker-bus conductors and drivers. This large sample of individuals also had the built-in variables that Morris needed to conduct his experiment. The conductors, or ticket takers, moved around during their work-day and climbed an average of 500 to 750 steps every day, while the drivers sat for over 90 percent of their shift. Morris surmised that the proof could be found on the stairs of those double-decker buses, which inspired him in 1949 to begin tracing the heart attack rates of hundreds of drivers and conductors. It may seem like a foregone conclusion for us today, but at the time, Morris's results astounded even him: the conductors had notably less coronary artery disease than the drivers, and if the conductors did develop disease, it happened much later on and was less likely to be fatal. Morris theorized that "physically active work" offered a protective effect, predominantly related to sudden cardiac death as a first manifestation of disease. He published his study in the prestigious *Lancet* medical journal, but it would go largely unnoticed and underappreciated for a long time. In the same paper, Morris and his team described similar findings in a group of 110,000 postal workers and civil servants. They clearly demonstrated that postmen who cycled or walked to deliver mail had fewer cardiac events when compared with workers engaged in less physical activity, from counter hands and postal supervisors to those who were a lot more sedentary such as telephone operators, civil service executives, and clerks.

As a further test of his hypothesis, Morris looked at how different social classes played into the risk for a heart attack and found more evidence to support his germinating theory. Regardless of social status, those people who engaged in the most active occupations enjoyed the benefit of a lower risk for cardiovascular disease. But it wasn't easy for Morris to get his message across to either his peers or to the masses. This early proposition that "men doing physically active work have a lower mortality from coronary heart disease in middle age than men in less active work" was met with "considerable skepticism by medical scientists and practitioners." His colleagues believed other factors were the chief reason for his results, such as socioeconomics and age, because it was just too unfathomable that physical activity alone could be such a powerful force. Morris persevered and continued to make his case. In the 1960s, he conducted an eight-year study of the overall physical activity of eighteen thousand men in sedentary civil service jobs. The data showed that those who engaged in regular aerobic exercise—fast walking, cycling, swimming, or other sports—reduced their risk of heart attack by half.

It took a couple of decades of painstaking work performed by not just Morris, but others equally curious and dedicated, to firmly prove the undeniable link between physical activity and heart health, and on the broader scale, physical activity and overall health. By the 1970s, people were beginning to take note and appreciate Morris's findings, including the International Olympic Committee, which awarded him its first prize in sports science in 1972. By the time Morris published another of his copious studies in 1980, more than thirty years after his first on the matter, he had valid proof that "vigorous exercise is a natural defense of the body, with a protective effect on the aging heart against ischemia and its consequences."

Today Morris is celebrated in scientific circles as the man who invented the field of physical-activity epidemiology, though he is barely known to the public. He was indefatigable in his efforts to promote public health and reduce health disparities. Morris was especially concerned with social equality and health and would describe himself as a "two-headed hedgehog." He continued his academic work and his passionate pursuit of knowledge to the end of his life, with eleven papers published in the scientific literature during his tenth decade. Morris stated it perfectly in 2009 when he wrote the following in a book: "We in the West are the first generation in human history in which the mass of the population has to deliberately exercise to be healthy. How can society's collective adaptations match?"

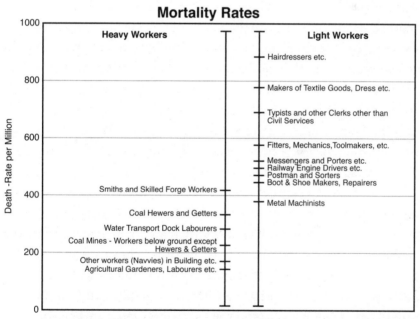

This figure was published in Morris's original paper in the *Lancet*, 1953. It shows the mortality rates from coronary heart disease among heavy and light workers, men aged forty-five to sixty-four in England and Wales from 1930 to 1932. The most sedentary jobs—such as that of the hairdresser (before chemicals were introduced!), typists, and those who primarily sat throughout the day—conferred the highest risk of heart attack, as seen on the right. The most laborious of jobs—those that had people primarily working hard outside—were associated with the lowest risk of dying from a heart attack. Today, we could envision a similar chart where construction workers and laborers would still be found on the lower left, and corporate executives and receptionists would be on the upper right. That is, unless those whose jobs revolve around computers and desks use their "leisure time" wisely—and actively.

Source: J.N. Morris et al. Coronary heart disease and physical activity of work. *Lancet* 2 (1953): 1053–57. Reprinted with permission.

Among the other visionaries who worked in Morris's footsteps was Ralph S. Paffenbarger, who shared the 1972 Olympic prize in sports science with Morris. Equally as charismatic and irrepressible as Morris, Paffenbarger added a few more important and cogent facts to the story of exercise, which would further help this new area of medicine gain a foothold in the general community. Paffenbarger was an American, born twelve years after Morris in Columbus, Ohio. He received a bachelor's degree from Ohio State University in 1944, and subsequently graduated from Northwestern University's medical school in 1947. He followed his medical education with a master's degree and then a doctorate in public health from Johns Hopkins University. At first, his research interests focused on preventive medicine and public health, and he spent time investigating one of the more pressing concerns of the era: polio. But by the mid-1950s, Jonas Salk had that problem pretty much solved with his polio vaccine, and Paffenbarger soon began focusing on physical activity as it relates to the development of diseases. He was one of the early investigators involved in the Framingham Heart Study, which laid the foundation for a great deal of cardiovascular disease studies that followed over the next decades. During this time he began to be interested in the possible role of physical inactivity in the development of cardiovascular disease. He would often talk about those early days and his conversations with individuals such as Paul Dudley White, the famous Boston cardiologist, and James Watt, the first director of the National Heart Institute. Shortly before Paffenbarger joined the National Heart Institute, he learned of Morris's London bus studies, which had just been published. Paffenbarger would later meet Morris, and the two would forge a friendship that lasted for the rest of their lives.

Like Morris before him, Paffenbarger looked into the associations between populations and their habits and compared them with longevity outcomes. Similar to Morris's studies that commenced in the 1950s, Paffenbarger made a name for himself beginning in the 1960s with two now-classic case studies: the College Alumni Health Study and the San Francisco Longshoremen Study. Both of these led to first-of-a-kind reports on topics such as physical activity and stroke, hypertension, diabetes, and longevity. In essence, they helped draw further conclusions about the kinds of things Morris was noticing in his own investigations.

What Paffenbarger proved so unmistakably was that independent of obesity, diet, and blood pressure, an inverse relationship exists between the amount of physical labor you do and your risk for heart disease and stroke. The less labor, the more risk you bear. This conclusion may seem like a duplicate of Morris's inferences, and in some ways it is. But Paffenbarger's work helped add more volume and dimension to the studies led by Morris, and it would come at a time when society, including its doubting, eternally questioning physicians, was better prepared to hear the news. Paffenbarger was also noted for his remarks on "leisure-time activities." In his Longshoreman Study, he had the benefit of watching technological advances on the docks that dramatically reshaped the physical demands of the workplace. At the beginning of the study (1951–60), 40 percent of longshoremen engaged in heavy work that proved to be protective for coronary heart disease mortality, but this declined to 15 percent by 1961–70, and only 5 percent by 1972. This led Paffenbarger to state, "If high energy output is protective, workers thus deprived of heavy work on the job may have to compensate by vigorous leisure-time activities, lest they encounter increased risk of fatal coronary heart."

Since many of us don't work in laborious jobs, "leisure-time activities" become essential. This is challenged by the competing demands of our digital world that make physical activity at work and at home in inevitable decline. During both Paffenbarger's and Morris's lives, our society began to undergo radical shifts in how we worked, commuted, and conducted our leisure-time activities—shifts that continue to this day with ever more ways to stay seated, stationary, and idle. Laborsaving devices were rare before World War II, but since then they have proliferated rapidly in both work settings and on the home front. From assembly-line machinery to appliances, automobiles, and electronics, we have an enormous array of ways to expend little energy in everyday pursuits. Both Morris and Paffenbarger commented on these circumstances over and over in their mission to establish a culture of exercise. They knew what they were up against—a culture increasingly finding excuses to remain sedentary—and they shared a fiery resolve to change social mores and public policy. A prime example of Morris's ability to convert complex phenomena into powerful messages is demonstrated in his often-quoted paper "Exercise in the Prevention of Coronary Heart Disease: Today's Best Buy in Public Health," which was published in 1994 when he was eighty-four years young.

The teaching that "some exercise is better than none, while more is better than some" may seem simplistic and obvious for us, but it took a breathtaking sixty-odd years of research before it was accepted. Even today, research continues based on the early principles established by these two men and that have since shaped governmental regulations, public policy, and, even more remarkably, the attitudes of millions of people. As this book went to press, a group of researchers led by Timothy S. Church at the Pennington Biomedical Research Center in Baton Rouge reported on a new study that blames our sizable weight gain in the general population on the sweeping shifts in the labor force since 1960. Jobs requiring moderate physical activity, including those in the agriculture and manufacturing, which accounted for 50 percent of the labor market in 1960, have dropped to just 20 percent. I don't think it's all that surprising to see a relationship between obesity and the lack of rigor of our jobs today. Church's latest conclusion simply adds to those already established by such people as Morris and Paffenbarger. It's unlikely that the lost physical activity can ever fully be restored to the workplace, but we can increase our physical activity outside work.

Paffenbarger himself was so moved by his studies from the get-go that he had to swallow some of his own medicine because he realized that a career in medicine deprived him of much-needed exercise. His finding that men who take up exercise later in life receive similar benefits to those enjoyed by lifelong exercisers motivated Paffenbarger, a previously sedentary man with a strong family history of premature coronary disease, to start running in the fall of 1967 at the age of forty-five. By 1993, when he was forced to retire from running at age seventy-one, he had competed in 151 marathons and ultramarathons, including twenty-two Boston Marathons and five grueling Western States 100 Endurance Runs—completing his first hundred-mile race through the Sierra Nevada in less than twenty-nine hours at the age of fifty-four. Don't panic: you don't need to be this ambitious about exercise to reap its benefits. What I'm going to advocate is much easier—and vastly less time-consuming—than this. Obviously, Paffenbarger was an anomaly in more ways than one, breaking new ground in and out of his office.

More than fifty years after Morris and Paffenbarger began their studies, they continued to express dissatisfaction with their colleagues in medicine, health care, and government for the limited degree to which they were translating the burgeoning evidence for the effects of exercise on health into meaningful clinical practice and public programs. They were your quintessential diehards, ruffling feathers, nagging, cajoling, prodding, and doing whatever it took to stimulate action on promoting physical activity. In a foreword to a book published in 2003, Morris could not resist stating: "In the half-century since the Second World War, there has been an explosion of research and thinking on the need for, and benefits of, physical activity/exercise across the lifespan and bodily systems. This knowledge is widely not being applied in practice. In consequence, there is an epochal waste of human potential for health, functional capacities, and well-being." In that same book, he writes, "When history comes to be written, society's failure to apply modern knowledge of normal ageing processes, in particular, the loss of muscle, and the remedial possibilities, is likely to shame us." I couldn't agree more with him.

Interestingly enough, Paffenbarger lived to be eighty-four years old, dying of heart failure in 2007; his comrade Morris lived to be ninety-nine and a half, dying also of heart failure, in 2009. According to his daughter, Morris always insisted on adding the "half." Morris kept up his own exercise habits for as long as possible; almost every day, well into his midnineties, he swam, pedaled his exercise bike, or walked for at least half an hour. Perhaps Morris and Paffenbarger bantered back and forth in their ripe old ages about whose body would give up first. Unlike so many other inquisitive thinkers who never get to see their ideas and work accepted by their peers and the world at large, it's nice to know that these two trailblazers got to witness the birth of the fitness movement, despite their ongoing frustrations with a lack of strong support from government institutions. The trends in aerobics, running, and formal events such as city marathons and triathlons would have to come from the people. And they did.

Exercise Physiology Takes Off

The story of exercise would not be complete without a nod to one more individual who is often the man credited for starting the fitness movement. He is Kenneth Cooper, and he introduced the concept of "aerobics" with the publication of his book by the same name in 1968. His book emphasized a point system for improving the cardiovascular system, which eventually became the basis of the ten thousand steps per day method of maintaining adequate fitness by walking. Cooper is the founder of the famous Cooper Aerobics Center in Dallas and McKinney, Texas, where scores of athletes have gone and continue to go to train for their events, including the Olympics. He is also the founder of the nonprofit research and education organization the Cooper Institute, which was opened in 1970.

Since the days of Morris's and Paffenbarger's early studies, which have become a symbol of a game-changing moment in the way we think about physical activity, exercise physiology has come a long way, especially in recent years. It's moved from an observational area of study to one that enjoys the advances we've made in the sciences to probe deeper into the whys and hows of the body's response to exercise from a biological standpoint. Some of this new knowledge has come from the wellness centers and research organizations established by Cooper, who, like Morris and Paffenbarger, has been a relentless promoter for physical activity, helping science debunk old myths that gave people excuses to stay put.

We know so much more about the mechanics of the human body through laboratory and clinical tests that show us exactly what's going on when we charge up a hill, take up power yoga, or just sit in front of a computer all day and relax on the couch at night. It's one thing to have anecdotal or population-based evidence of the health advantages that exercise can afford us, but it's clearly another to have hard data to help explain the biochemical facts—from how our blood work changes to even how the expression of our genes swings in different directions. Under the umbrella of exercise physiology, entire new fields of medicine have been created, and thousands of studies are published now each year in this subject. Take a look at the following figure, which vividly showcases the swift increase in studies examining the link between physical activity, fitness, and cardiovascular disease. It was published in the *Annals of Epidemiology* within a commemorative article written as a tribute to Jeremiah Morris upon his death. Check out the difference just between the 1990s and 2000s. It's remarkable to think we've more than doubled our investigations into these matters of fitness health in only the last decade or so.

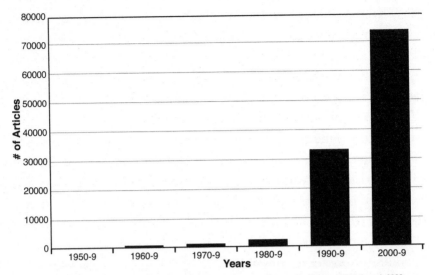

Number of published articles on physical activity, fitness, and cardiovascular disease—1950 through 2009.
Web of Science search terms: "physical activity or physical fitness and cardiovascular disease or coronary
heart disease." Number of articles in each time interval: 142; 493; 1,083; 2,939; 33,932; and 74,162 respectively.
Source: S.N. Blair et al. A tribute to Professor Jeremiah Morris: the man who invented the field of physical activity epidemiology.
Annals of Epidemiology 20, no. 9 (September 2010): 651–60. Reprinted with permission.

One of the hottest subbranches of exercise physiology today, or,
as some would say, physical-activity epidemiology, is metabolomics,
a form of metabolic profiling that aims to find biochemical patterns
in people that either spell disease or lower their risk for certain illnesses. Metabolomics has given us a window into the connection
between being fit and having a fit metabolism that not only burns
calories efficiently but also helps us to maintain that all-important
homeostasis that I've been talking about. This is due to metabolic
changes that occur during exercise and keep our body on an even,
self-regulating keel. One case in point: Fit people in a study done
by a team from the Massachusetts General Hospital and the Broad
Institute of MIT and Harvard were found to have greater increases
in a metabolite called niacinamide than unfit people. Niacinamide
is a nutrient by-product that's involved with blood-sugar control.
In fact, this team found more than twenty metabolites that change
during exercise. These are naturally produced compounds that help

burn calories and fat and improve blood-sugar control. Some weren't known until now to be involved with exercise. Some revved up during exercise, such as those helping to process fat. Other compounds involved with cellular stress decreased with exercise.

There's no end to the number of studies that prove the power of exercise in maintaining health, and I trust that we'll see this body of research continue to grow. In 2009 another study emerged clearly showing evidence that exercise causes your brain to boost production of certain chemicals known to have antidepressant effects. Anything that helps us stave off depression and cultivate happiness is good for health. The researchers also discovered that exercise excited a gene for a nerve growth factor called VGF. VGFs are small proteins critical to the development and maintenance of nerve cells, which further links exercise to brain health and the prevention of dementia and Alzheimer's disease. Even more fascinating, the study brought to light thirty-three VGFs that show altered activity with exercise, the majority of which had never before been identified. Maybe someday we'll uncover the direct relationship between these molecular changes and the prevention of cancer and other illnesses that reflect breakdowns in the system. The anecdotal evidence is already there.

On a more basic level, people forget the effects that aging has on our bodies and abilities to maintain a strong metabolism. In addition to the muscle loss and strength that we experience naturally alongside the inevitable slowdown of our metabolisms over time, we fail to consider the practical reasons for weight gain: we tend to become more sedentary yet don't change our eating habits. Hormonal changes hammer more nails in the coffin, exacerbating an already troubled metabolism. A study released in 2010 and published in the *Journal of the American Medical Association* stated clearly that the 2008 US guidelines urging about a half hour of exercise five days a week won't stop weight gain in older people if they do not cut calories. It takes more effort and time to lose more as we age more. The research is more sobering for those who are already overweight:

227

even more exercise is called for to avoid gaining weight without eating less.

Can exercise physically *reverse* aging? Stalling or slowing down aging is one thing, but what about literally (and obviously physiologically) shifting it into a reverse gear? This question has sparked exploration of another exciting area, and though it may sound like science fiction, we already have some proof to consider. In 2008 a team of Canadian and American researchers showed that exercise can partially help reverse aging at the cellular level. They looked at the effects of six months of strength training in elderly volunteers aged sixty-five and older, taking small biopsies of thigh-muscle cells from the seniors before and after the six months. The researchers then compared the cells with muscle cells from twenty-six young volunteers whose average age was twenty-two. The scientists expected to find evidence that the program improved the seniors' strength, which it did by 50 percent; but they were quite bewildered by the dramatic changes they found in gene expression. The gene expression in the muscle-cell fingerprint of the elderly volunteers who'd gone through the strength-training program was reversed nearly to that of younger people. In other words, their muscle gene-expression profile resembled that of a younger group.

This may seem like a strange and difficult thing to "see" and measure from a scientific standpoint, but we have all the technology to perform such amazing experiments today. What these researchers did was compare the expression of six hundred genes found in muscles both at the beginning of the six-month period and then at the end. They found significant differences between the older and younger participants in the expression of these genes, indicating that these genes become either more or less active with age. By the end of the exercise phase, the expression of a third of those genes had changed, and upon closer observation the researchers realized that the ones that changed were the genes involved in the functioning of mitochondria. Mitochondria are tiny organelles within cells that combine oxygen and nutrients to create fuel for the cells; they are our cells' chief energy generators. This research has since been confirmed by other noteworthy studies.

Many scientists consider the loss of healthy mitochondria to be an important underlying cause of aging in mammals. Mitochondria have their own DNA, distinct from the cell's own genetic material, and they multiply on their own. But mitochondria can accumulate small genetic mutations, which under normal circumstances are corrected by specialized repair systems within the cell. Over time, as we age, the number of mutations begins to outstrip the system's ability to make repairs, and mitochondria start malfunctioning and dying. As our mitochondria falter, the cells they fuel wither or die. The results are the hallmarks of aging as muscles shrink, brain volume drops, hair falls out or becomes gray, and soon enough we are, in appearance and beneath the surface, old. Experiments in mice have shown that the ones that exercise maintain healthy mitochondria and clearly outlive their sedentary counterparts. They also age much better.

What Smoking and Sitting Have in Common (Even If You Don't Smoke)

So what should we be doing? Ideally, a well-rounded and comprehensive exercise program includes cardio work, strength training, and stretching. Each of these activities affords us unique benefits that our body needs to achieve and maintain peak performance, and, apparently, to affect our genes and metabolism. Cardio work, which gets the heart rate up for an extended period, will burn calories, lower body fat, and strengthen both the heart and lungs; strength training (use of weights or elastic bands, or even your own body weight as resistance) will keep your bones strong and prevent that loss of lean muscle mass; and stretching will keep you flexible and less susceptible to joint pain and that dreaded condition of chronic inflammation.

Also don't forget that the benefits of exercise are cumulative. Science has proven, from origins in Morris's and Paffenbarger's work, that short exercise bouts throughout the day are just as effective as one long workout and may be even *better*. "Interval training" may be all the rage today, but it's been documented for decades. When Paffenbarger looked at the effects of "repeated bursts of work activity" in 6,351 longshoremen way back in 1975, which is the old-fashioned way of saying interval training, he noted that repeated bursts of high-energy output had a protective effect on their hearts, lowering their risk for disease.

The essence of interval training is going hard for a short period, then backing off for a few minutes before resuming a higher level of intensity for another short interval. You can do this in virtually any type of exercise, from walking to utilizing equipment in a gym. Modifying your speed, adding weights, or trying hills of varying steepness are all ways in which you can create your own interval training routine.

Spreading your workouts throughout the day into short bursts has another benefit: it helps prevent you from the ravages that sitting down for long periods of time can do to your body. Researchers at the American Cancer Society released a study published in 2010 in the *American Journal of Epidemiology* that pretty much said sitting down for extended periods poses a health risk as "insidious" as smoking or overexposure to the sun. The people in the study were followed from 1993 to 2006; researchers examined their amount of time spent sitting and their physical activity in relation to mortality over the thirteen years. A second study at the International Diabetes Institute in Melbourne concluded that even two hours of exercise a day would not compensate for "spending 22 hours sitting on your rear end."

While several studies support a link between sitting time and obesity, type 2 diabetes, cardiovascular disease, and unhealthy dietary patterns, few studies have examined time spent sitting in relation to total mortality. This latest study makes a stunning case for the strong association between continually sitting down (as many of us do nowadays at desks, on the couch, and in our cars) and disease. The unfair shocker: women seem to be more affected by spending time on their derrieres. In the study, women who reported more than six hours per day of sitting (outside of work) were 37 percent more likely to die during the time period studied than those who sat fewer than three hours a day. Men who sat more than six hours a day (also outside of work) were 18 percent more likely to die than those who sat fewer than three hours per day. The association remained virtually unchanged after adjusting for physical activity level.

Sitting itself is not the culprit here, it's the biological effects that sitting triggers in the body. Just as exercise spurs positive metabolic changes to our system, sedentariness causes metabolic changes in the opposite, negative direction. And prolonged time spent sitting, *independent of physical activity*, has been shown to have significant metabolic consequences, influencing such things as triglycerides, cholesterol, blood sugar, resting blood pressure, and the appetite hormone leptin, all of which are risk factors for obesity, cardiovascular illness, and other chronic diseases.

What's more, yet another study published just this year shared similar findings. Researchers from the Department of Epidemiology and Public Health at the University College London reported that spending in excess of four hours a day sitting in front of a television or computer more than doubles your risk of dying from or being hospitalized for heart disease. Even those who exercise can't overcome the detrimental effects of prolonged inactivity. In this study, the researchers found that blood levels of C-reactive protein, that marker of inflammation, were twice as high in people who spent more than four hours in front of a screen than people who spent fewer than two.

That we tend to overestimate how much we actually move throughout the day hit home for me when a company sent me an accelerometer to test out. Prior to that experiment, I thought I was an active person during the day, even though most of my day is spent in the office. This nifty little device had a small microchip that tracked my movement as I wore it on my belt for several weeks and reviewed the data on my computer. It recorded that for hours at a time I was on conference calls and not moving. I was actually surprised at my sedentariness and quickly bought a wireless telephone headset that I now wear like headphones, which enables me to walk around while I talk. This one tiny change made a big difference, as I was able to increase the number of steps I took in a day at work by 35 percent!

The message is clear: we must move—and move frequently—to maintain health. Unless you're an old-fashioned longshoreman or trolley conductor, which I doubt any of you are, then take heed. It's not just a matter of fitness. It's a matter of life and longevity. Don't make the mistake in thinking that exercise is only good for heart health, either. I may have said a lot about the benefits that physical activity offers the cardiovascular system, but I should reiterate that exercise is good for all of your systems. To summarize every single major study of late that demonstrates the profound and irrefutable connection between exercise and virtually all other types of diseases and disorders, including degenerative and autoimmune disease, and cancer, I would need to write another book. So just remember the bottom line: exercise is the only proven fountain of youth that doesn't require a pill or potion; and being physically fit does a body's complex system good.

For those of you who need to be convinced of this recommendation in a more visual manner, check out the following figure, which was published in 2009 in the *British Journal of Sports Medicine* (Morris would be proud). In a nutshell, it shows that having a "low cardiorespiratory fitness," or low CRF, which is really code for being out of shape, accounts for a greater proportion of deaths than any of the other conditions listed, including obesity, diabetes, or high cholesterol, and it even beats out the smoker. Hypertension in men is the only condition that comes close to the ravages of low fitness.

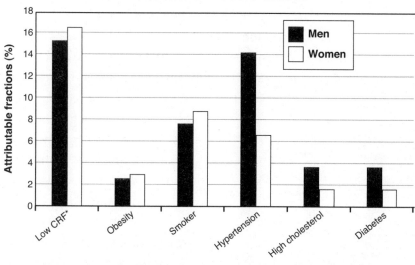

Men/Women Causes of Death

Attributable fractions (%) for all-cause deaths in 40,842 (3,333 deaths) men and 12,943 (491 deaths) women in the Aerobics Center Longitudinal Study. The attributable fractions are adjusted for age and each other item in the figure. *Cardiorespiratory fitness determined by a maximal exercise test on a treadmill.

Source: S.N. Blair et al. A tribute to Professor Jeremiah Morris: the man who invented the field of physical activity epidemiology. *Annals of Epidemiology*, 20, no. 9 (September 2010): 651–60. Reprinted with permission.

Even people who just break up their sitting time by walking around with a free weight to perform a few biceps curls can lower their risk of disease and premature death. I'd suggest you keep a pair of 2.5-pound weights by your desk, under your couch, and anywhere you spend time. Stand on one foot and do twenty reps while on your next phone call with a headset; this is a great abdominal exercise that also helps you work on your balance.

Whether it's a structured class at a gym, power walking with friends in the morning, dancing, or streaming videos over the Internet with the latest from fitness trainers, you have lots of options to stay in shape today. I must repeat: you don't need to sign up for an athletic event, invest in a home gym, or even join a traditional gym. The type of activity you do is not nearly as important as how often you do it, how long you do it, and performing varied intervals. Just pick something you love! Exercise should be enjoyable, and something you look forward to every day. Life is a marathon rather than an all-out sprint, and your workouts should reflect that.

A couple of extra pointers: (1) because exercise has been shown to lower stress for up to twenty-four hours, it's important to avoid being the "weekend warrior" and to keep a daily routine with an occasional day of rest and recovery; and (2) it's also not a good idea to go much past an hour, especially if you're determined to push your boundaries and challenge yourself physically. The benefits of exercise begin to diminish when you exceed an hour, and at that point you could be harming the body more than you're protecting it. (I won't get into the pros and cons of endurance training and speak to the marathoners and triathletes out there; I'll save that for another time.)

> Minimum goal: get your heart rate up 50 percent for at least fifteen minutes every day. Design your day for you and your health. Limit exercises that focus on and isolate certain muscle groups, as these can be prescriptions for back pain, neck pain, etc., later on. If you don't feel well one day, still aim to engage in some exercise barring any serious illness or fever. Remember, consistency is the key, but you should also get creative and have fun with your activity. Don't make exercise a chore, and don't make yourself miserable by doing something you hate.

As with your diet, don't be dishonest about your efforts. While surveys show that nearly a third of people consider themselves "very active," the obesity numbers indicate otherwise. The true number of people who get an hour of moderate exercise every day has been estimated closer to an abysmal 5 percent. Many forms of exercise can involve your family and friends, which can be motivating and offer an added benefit—especially psychologically. Giving yourself consistent low-impact recovery days is also part of a well-rounded workout routine.

Routines don't only relate to regular workout regimens. Routines of all sorts, as you're about to find out, have everything to do with health. Life might seem repetitious and mechanical in a lot of ways from day to day, but that's how your body likes it—more than you would ever believe.

Health Rule

Sitting for long periods of time, even if you exercise rigorously once during the day, has biologic effects that are surprisingly worse than we ever imagined. Find opportunities to move your body as much as you can during the course of your usual day. For example, take the stairs instead of the elevator, and get a cordless telephone to walk around your office while speaking rather than sit at your desk. All of this should be in addition to engaging in traditional exercise.

11

Timing Is Everything

The Wonder Drug of Keeping a Regular Schedule

A s you can imagine, I get a lot of calls from people who fear they have cancer. Fatigue and a vague feeling that something "isn't right" are their chief complaints, and they want me to figure out what's wrong with them. They ask me to ease their worry that cancer isn't to blame for their apparent malaise. Unfortunately, there's no single test I can perform for a definitive diagnosis, or even to see if cells are doing something suspicious in an organ or tissue. Although people would like to think I can throw them into a scanner or draw some blood to make immediate sense of their low energy, I have to tell them the truth: it's not that simple. A battery of traditional tests can clue me in to a few things, but they won't necessarily tell me what people want—or don't want—to hear. In the future, hopefully we'll have better, more precise diagnostics that can solve this kind of mystery quickly and cheaply. But for now the answer often hinges on old-fashioned sleuthing that's more of an art than a science.

First, I ask them about their daily habits. What does their day

look like? How much do they sleep? What did they eat for break-
fast? How has their routine or schedule changed recently? What
medications and supplements do they take? The artistry of my job
begins as I try to decode the puzzle.

Some of these patients do have some cancering going on, but
many don't. To recapture their energy and sense of well-being, all
I have to prescribe for them is a few basic guidelines, the common
denominator of which is keeping a *regular schedule*. That means paying attention to when they sleep, when they eat, when they exercise,
and how they manage stress. Which is actually not so easy to do
in today's hyperkinetic world of 24-7 activity. It's difficult to con-
ceive the significance that keeping a regular schedule can have on us
physiologically and emotionally until we are robbed of that reliable
regimen. Most of us know what it's like to lose a few nights' sleep
over a deadline at work, or after traveling long distances across time
zones; our bodies feel "off" and we're not likely to rank our energy
levels at a perfect 10 as we try to adapt to a modified schedule. We
eat differently. We don't stick to the same exercise routine (or we
skip it entirely). We may do things at unusual times such as eat lunch
really late or sleep in to make up for another long night at the office.

Another way to think about this is to recall the last time you were
sick with a dreadful cold or stomach bug. You may have spent some
time sleeping in bed during the day when you're normally up and
about. When we're ill, we're more irregular than when we're healthy,
and we may even comfort ourselves with certain foods we wouldn't
normally eat as a way of "enduring" the illness. It's interesting that during times of stress, be it related to work or suffering a passing bug, we
tend to throw our schedules far off when we should really be going in
the other direction—maintaining the stricter schedule that our bodies
prefer, and choosing the most nutrient-packed foods per calorie.

There's a reason you wake up at exactly the same time every
morning even on days you wish to sleep in; there's a reason your
kids cry when you're a half hour late serving them a meal. When

you break the body's natural rhythm, you're no longer performing optimally—your state has been disrupted. To be healthy, you must respect and maintain that ideal, rhythmic state.

Perhaps the greatest demonstration of the influence our schedules can have on us is found in the difference between grievers and dog walkers. Grief is a proven killer. Numerous studies have shown that people who are grieving following the loss of a close loved one bear a higher risk of dying. A lot of that risk, however, isn't necessarily tied to the emotional pull of surviving a loss, which can affect the body physically. Indeed, dying of a "broken heart" does have its stress-related underpinnings; people have been known to drop dread of a heart attack upon hearing devastating news or on the anniversary of a stressful event. In these cases, a person's emotional state, operating at a subconscious level, can interact with serious preexisting heart disease to trigger a cardiac event. But for grievers who experience prolonged mourning, something else goes on that ups their mortality. They become irregular with their daily schedules as they grieve, from what time they get up and go to bed to what they choose to eat and how they move their bodies. They no longer keep to the same old routines while they struggle to adapt to a new status quo, which can entail new living arrangements in the case of a widow or widower. This disorganized, erratic, and chaotic management of their time and habits can have more destructive repercussions than they realize.

Let's take one universal habit as an example. If you were to step into a body that's been deprived of its expectation of eating at a certain time, you'd witness events going on that would likely surprise you. Take, for instance, the mundane habit of eating lunch. If you consistently eat at one o'clock in the afternoon, and one day an unexpected phone call or obligation has you postponing your lunch until much later, say two or three, your body won't just show signs of hunger in that waiting period. It will also experience a surge in cortisol, the stress hormone that tells our bodies to hold tightly to fat and to conserve energy. The body, in essence, goes into survival mode because it's suddenly unable to predict when it will get its next meal. Of all the things that a body loves, predictability is one of them. One of the biggest components of stress for our bodies is not our finances, our marriages, or the kids—it's regularity of schedule or lack thereof.

Small changes in schedule can have profound effects on how we feel and the stress level of our body. The take-home message is to eat at regular times, whether it be three or five meals a day. The number of meals means little compared with the regularity of when you eat. So, the people who grab an apple or granola bar whenever they feel hungry are doing themselves a big disservice. Having a snack every day at 3:00 p.m. is the better approach and has markedly different effects on the body than the random snacking.

Recall what I explained earlier about the body's need for homeostasis, which is constancy in the face of environmental fluctuations. The whole point of regulation is to maintain the body in a relatively constant state. Yes, it's dynamic and changing all the time, but the body perpetually modifies itself to create the steadiness that it craves—to stay in a zone where it's safe and protected from harm. If you think about it, the body is perpetually under forces that work against constancy, such as your choosing when to eat and what time you'll surrender to sleep and go to bed. Even the temperature of your environment keeps your body working to maintain a steady 98.6 degrees Fahrenheit. What we often don't think about, however, is what our bodies actually do from a biochemical standpoint when we don't follow its preferred rhythms, and when its preferred rhythms cannot stay streamlined.

It's hard to imagine the omnipotent pull that schedules and routines can have on human health, but a look at what's been going on in the sleep-medicine community provides an enlightening window. Of all the things that sleep patterns do to affect our lives, one of the most commanding roles they have is their ability to dictate our hormonal balance. This hormonal balance in turn affects a wide variety of processes in the body that are part of our overall health equation.

ur Body Balanced

e's multiple benefits that are written about daily in
you're paying attention), sleep has similarly shared
time in the nelight lately because of its numerous pro-health effects on the body. Both laboratory and clinical studies have shown
that virtually every system in the body is affected by the quality and
amount of sleep we get a night. Among the proven benefits: sleep
can dictate how much we eat, how fast our metabolisms run, how
fat or thin we get, whether we can fight off infections, how creative
and insightful we can be, how well we can cope with stress, how
quickly we can process information and learn new things, and how
well we can organize and store memories. Losing as few as one and a
half hours that our body needs for just one night can reduce daytime
alertness by about a third. The side effects of poor sleep habits are
many: hypertension, confusion, memory loss, the inability to learn
new things, obesity, cardiovascular disease, and depression.

While many of us have a sense of our hormonal cycles, women
especially, throughout our lives, we don't all appreciate how those
cycles feed into our sense of well-being and hinge largely on sleep
habits. Michael Breus is one of this country's leading figures in sleep medicine. In his book *Good Night*, he describes in detail just how essential sleep is in our lives, emphasizing what it ultimately gives us: steady homeostatic states. We all have a biological internal clock called a circadian rhythm, men included. It's defined by the patterns of repeated activity associ-

We don't establish a circadian rhythm until about six weeks of age. That's about the time when babies can hold more milk in their tummies to sleep for longer periods. While most infants take longer to adjust to sleeping through the night, any parent who's been lucky to have a newborn sleep through the night at such a young age can thank those rhythms that begin ticking and will tick their whole lives.

ated with the environmental cycles of day and night—rhythms that recur roughly every twenty-four hours. Examples include our sleep-wake cycle, the ebb and flow of certain biochemicals, the rise and fall of body temperature, and other subtle rhythms that mesh with the twenty-four-hour solar day. When our rhythm is not in sync with the twenty-four-hour solar day, we'll feel out of sorts. Anyone who has traveled across time zones and felt off-kilter for a few days can understand this.

So much of our body's natural rhythm revolves around our sleep habits. Normal hormonal secretion patterns—from those that govern our eating behaviors to those that help us fight illness and manage stress—are tied directly to the health of our day/night cycles. Cortisol, for example, should peak in the morning and progressively decrease throughout the day, dipping to its lowest levels after 11:00 p.m., at which point melatonin levels are high. Melatonin, as many of you know, is our sleep hormone. But it actually helps regulate our entire twenty-four-hour rhythm as well. Once released after the sun sets, it slows body function, lowers blood pressure, and in turn core body temperature so we're prepared to sleep. Higher melatonin levels will allow for more deep sleep, which helps maintain healthy levels of growth hormone, thyroid hormone, and male and female sex hormones. Some studies have even hinted that shift workers, people with the most erratic sleep schedules, may live with a high risk for certain cancers.

The commanding role that biological rhythms play in our sense of well-being and level of physical power and alertness explains why studies done on people throughout their day show performance can be linked to the time of day. Is there an ideal time to serve a really fast tennis ball? Indeed, at 6:00 p.m., when the body's temperature and grip strength are highest. What about swimming four hundred meters in your best Olympic imitation? The evening hours can again give us a slight advantage over the early morning. Our body temperature goes up during the day, peaks in the evening, then begins to go down again, bottoming out sometime in the early-morning hours. It also takes a slight dip in the early afternoon, which brings on that after-lunch lull. Exposure to bright light, especially from sunlight, helps naturally reset our rhythm every day so our sleep-wake cycles remain stable. Physical activity can act like light in this regard, too, helping set and maintain our biological clock naturally.

Sleep and hormones go hand in hand in ways many of us under-appreciate, and one in particular actually requires sleep to get re-leased. About twenty to thirty minutes after we first close our eyes, our pituitary gland at the base of our brain begins to pulsate out growth hormone. It will do this throughout the night during our deepest sleep cycle, but this first release is our body's highest level in a single day. Growth hormone does more than just stimulate cellular recovery and growth; it affects almost every cell in the body, renew-ing the skin and bones, regenerating the heart, liver, lungs, and kid-neys, and bringing back organ and tissue function to more youthful levels. It also revitalizes the immune system, lowers the risk factors of heart attack and stroke, improves oxygen uptake, and helps pre-vent osteoporosis. It even aids in our ability to maintain an ideal weight, effectively telling our cells to switch from using carbs for energy and to use fat instead.

In chapter 2, I noted how some men try to tap a fountain of youth by injecting themselves with human growth hormone. After all, given all the benefits I just attributed to this superhormone, it's logi-cal to think it could be sold as a supplement or used as an antiaging drug. New research, however, is pointing to the potential down-side to this trend: artificially boosting your levels of growth hor-mone could put you at higher risk for diabetes and cancer. So while human growth hormone is required in higher amounts during one's fast-developing youth, the body's system may not like (nor need) an excess supply later in life. It throws the system off somewhere. Find-ings like this emphasize the power of trade-offs in medicine. Yes, growth hormone can help make an older man feel like a teenager again and allow him to more easily build muscle mass, but it will have repercussions elsewhere in the body—and affect it in ways we don't yet understand. There's a reason the body doesn't produce the same volume of growth hormone in a seventy-year-old as in a seven-year-old. Also, a shot of growth hormone doesn't have the same effect on your system as a secretion that's naturally controlled by the circadian rhythm, which is timed to other bodily functions. We don't have a means to imitate how the body controls these hormones!

Sleep Is a Sentinel of a Healthy State

I have found that many people don't like to be told that sleep is arguably the easiest way to regulate their bodies and feel a positive difference in a short time. They don't want to believe me because they'd rather take a shortcut and pop a pill than be told to sleep better. But it's true: sleep directs so much of our body's hormonal rhythms and cycles that we can't just reboot ourselves artificially. We need a regular, reliable pattern of wakefulness and rejuvenating sleep to achieve that reboot and to regulate our hormones. This piece of advice doesn't hit home for many, though, until I remind them about the appetite hormones that hinge largely on sleep habits.

Ghrelin and leptin are science-speak for "eat" and "don't eat" respectively. You may have heard about these two digestive hormones in the media lately because a lot of attention has been placed on them following recent research. They are the yin and yang of our eating patterns, essentially telling us when we're hungry and when it's time to push away from the table. As with many hormones, these two are paired together but have opposing functions. Ghrelin (your "go" hormone) gets secreted by the stomach when it's empty and increases our appetite. It sends a message to our brain that we need to eat; it's our accelerator. When our stomach is full, fat cells usher out the other hormone—leptin—so our brain gets the message that we are full and need to stop eating. Leptin is our brake. The science that has made ghrelin and leptin so popular lately is that it's been proven that a bad night's sleep—or just not enough sleep—creates an imbalance of both hormones. When people snooze just four hours a night for two nights, they experience a 20 percent drop in leptin and an increase in ghrelin. They also have a marked increase (about 24 percent) in hunger and appetite, driving them toward calorie-dense, high-carbohydrate foods such as sweets, salty snacks, and starchy foods. Sleep deprivation essentially disconnects our brain from our stomach, leading to "mindless eating." It deceives our body into believing it's hungry (when it's not), and it also tricks us into craving foods that can spoil a healthy diet.

In addition to sleep habits, our environment, dietary habits, exercise patterns, personal stress levels, and our genetics may also influence the production of leptin and ghrelin. Though we don't know the exact ways in which these factors influence those hormones, this shows how many biological factors contribute to our behaviors, which in turn influence how we feel about what we do (or don't do). When we consider the parallels between our obesity epidemic and collective sleep deprivation, we have to wonder, can sleep be the ultimate diet? Sixty-five percent of Americans are overweight or obese, a percentage that takes on a special significance when an estimated 63 percent of American adults do not get the recommended eight hours of sleep a night. The average adult gets 6.9 hours of sleep on weeknights and 7.5 hours on weekends, for a daily average of seven hours.

Several epidemiological studies have demonstrated the connection between obesity and sleep. One such study, from Columbia University in New York, used government data on 6,115 people to compare sleep patterns and obesity. Researchers found that people who sleep two to four hours a night are 73 percent more likely to be obese than those who get seven to nine hours. Those who get five or more hours of sleep a night are 50 percent more likely to be obese than normal sleepers. Those who sleep six hours are 23 percent more likely to be obese; those who get 10 or more hours are 11 percent less likely to be obese.

This may seem, on the surface, counterintuitive to how we think. Most people assume that sleeping too much contributes to making people fat, but all the studies point to the opposite's being true. The reasoning makes sense: sleep-deprived people eat more because they're hungrier, they're awake longer, and they may be tempted by foods everywhere they go. They often consume far more calories than they burn in the extra hours they're awake. People are usually pretty sedentary in that extra waking time, engaging in "low-calorie" leisure activities such as watching TV, reading, surfing the Internet, and responding to e-mail. They may burn an extra fifty calories or so in several hours, but the changes in hormones prompt them to eat far more than fifty calories. The changes in their appetite regulation are way in excess of the calories needed for the extra hours of wakefulness.

Volumes of research now prove that, in addition to the hormones associated with eating, and ultimately weight control, irregular swings in cortisol are linked to depression. And irregular secretions of cortisol throughout the day can happen as a result of irregular sleeping patterns. This is yet another condition the shares a parallel universe with the obesity epidemic. Depression is on course to have a huge impact on our world in the near future. The World Health Organization has estimated that by the year 2020, depression will be the second-leading disability-causing disease in the world. In many developed countries, such as the United States, depression is already among the top causes of disability and mortality.

Your Internal HMO

Our body's ache for regularity has its survivalist origins. If we could cast back to millions of years ago and visit our ancestral cavemen and cavewomen, we'd find that a particular organ responsible for all this rhythmic regularity functions exactly the same now as it did then. That organ is your hypothalamus, and it's where your inner reptile lives. An exceedingly ancient structure that sits in the middle of your head, the hypothalamus is unlike most other more sophisticated and advanced brain regions and has maintained a striking similarity in structure throughout the course of human evolution. We'd even find remarkable similarities in the hypothalamus of animals that came long before mammals roamed the earth.

It was around the time of the dinosaurs, in fact, when this part of the brain evolved. No wonder the hypothalamus is so old: one of its main purposes is to beat starvation. In the absence of food, the hypothalamus releases biological chemicals that change how the body functions so it can find food to survive. For example, when faced with life-threatening starvation, the hypothalamus will trigger the release of a hormone called orexia, which, in tiny doses, can have far-reaching effects. It will make you acutely more alert, increase your capacity to engage your muscles to move, and heighten problem-solving so you can find food quickly.

This isn't all the hypothalamus can do; it helps to think of this ancient organ as the health maintenance organization of our entire body, a kind of headquarters for maintaining the body's preferred status quo—that crucial homeostasis or "balance." It houses several important centers that preside over a wide range of our physiology, including body temperature, thirst, water balance, circadian rhythms such as your sleep-wake cycles, fatigue, escape from danger, contractions during childbirth, and even arousal and sexual function. We owe our experiences of pleasure, aggression, stress, embarrassment, and aversion to our hypothalamus. It's fully functional when we are born, and one of its most important jobs is to link the nervous system to the hormonal system. This is possible through the help of the pituitary gland, a pea-size structure that dangles off the bottom of the hypothalamus. The pituitary usually steals all the credit for being the master hormonal gland because it's the one who sends out those behavior-altering hormones. But it does so at the command of the hypothalamus. It is the consummate servant to the hypothalamus.

I bring up the hypothalamus because one of the ways in which we can keep it healthy is by paying attention to our sleep habits. Poor sleep catches up to most of us. It also sets us up for entering a vicious cycle whereby we plunge into deeper sleep deprivation and drive our hypothalamus into overdrive, which can then sabotage all sorts of biological functions. Maintaining healthy sleep habits, what sleep doctors call sleep hygiene, can act as a center of gravity for ensuring your body stays balanced and homeostatic. It's actually easier to do than you think, but most people focus on the wrong aspect of sleep. Contrary to what you may believe, achieving restful sleep is not so much about the number of hours you bank each night. It's about something else.

The Magic Number

The body doesn't require a magic number of sleep hours. The amount of sleep you get also isn't as critical as you'd think. It's *regularity* of sleep that's important. Everyone has a different sleep need. The "eight-hour" rule is general, but not necessarily the ideal number for you. Most people need seven to nine hours at specific times during the twenty-four-hour day (e.g., 10:00 p.m. to 6:00 a.m.), and chances are you know what your metrics are. Despite what many people attempt to do, shifting your sleep habits on the weekends to "catch up" can disrupt a healthy circadian rhythm. Going to bed at 9:00 p.m. one night and 10:00 p.m. the next will similarly disrupt your natural cycle—even if you sleep for the same number of hours both nights.

As previously noted, the body is an amazing self-regulator. You can train yourself to sleep eight hours a night if you treat the body right by going to bed and getting up at the same time every day, week-

For a long time, we didn't think regular sleep could really improve athletic performance all that much, but now the proof is spilling out of labs the world over. Two such intriguing studies to note: One, from researchers at Stanford University, found that extra hours of sleep at night can help improve football players' performance on drills such as the forty-yard dash and what's called the twenty-yard shuttle. In Australia, researchers documented remarkable differences in performance when its national netball team (netball is a variation of the basketball theme) traveled across two time zones, thereby affecting regular sleep patterns.

ends included. People who can get by on just five hours a night are likely achieving the same amount of deep, restful sleep as those who sleep longer, but the time spent in the different stages of sleep is shorter.

Not surprisingly, stress and staying up too late are the two big culprits responsible for poor sleep, which is why it's important to establish a healthy sleep hygiene—the habits that make for a restful night's sleep regardless of factors such as age and underlying medical conditions that can disrupt sleep. The goal is to minimize those factors' effects on us so we can welcome peaceful sleep. In addition to the tips I've already given, here are a few more that will help you get a good night's sleep*:

- This one bears repeating: stick to the same sleep-wake schedule seven days a week. Even when you have a late night, get up at your usual time. Regularity—not total hours of sleep—is the key.
- Avoid napping if you don't usually nap on a regular, consistent basis. On the other hand, if you do main-

---

*For more ideas on regulating your sleep and even using sleep to lose weight, check out Michael Breus's website at www.thesleepdoctor.com and his latest book *The Sleep Doctor's Diet Plan*.

tain a regular routine of napping every day, then by all means stick with it.

- Set aside at least thirty minutes before bedtime to unwind and prepare for sleep. Avoid stimulating activities (e.g., work, fussing over undone chores, cleaning, being on the computer, watching TV dramas) that get your adrenaline running.
- Try to keep distracting electronics and gadgets out of the bedroom and maintain a tidy, cool, and dark environment. It should be your sleeping sanctuary.
- Cut back on caffeine in the afternoon, especially after 2:00. Your body needs time to process all the caffeine so it won't infringe upon restful sleep. If you cannot go cold turkey, then at least switch to drinks with less caffeine, such as teas.
- Be cautious about alcohol intake in the evening hours. A glass or two of wine within hours of bedtime will change how you sleep. You might want to test out avoiding any alcohol for a few days and see if it changes how refreshed you feel the next day.
- Keep your wakeful life on a relatively stable track. Exercise at the same time each day if you can. Eat meals as the same time. If you find yourself having to push your lunch to the later side, have a nutritious snack on hand and eat it when you would have had lunch. Give your body what it expects on a regular basis!

When to Consider a Sleep Aid

Is there ever an appropriate time to visit the medicine cabinet before bed? From over-the-counter remedies to prescriptions marketed as nonaddictive and safe, sleep aids are a gigantic industry. I'm all for using a sleep aid when necessary, such as recovering from a long business trip and getting back into the swing of things at home in my time zone. But user beware: Modern sleep medications may not be as chemically addicting as earlier generations of sleep drugs, but they can be psychologically addicting. They can prevent you from reaching the farthest reaches of deep sleep for long enough to reap all of its rewards. They may also make you feel groggy or "hungover" the next day.

Your doctor can help you rule out any underlying medical condition that could be robbing you of restful sleep. Sleep apnea, for instance, is common today mostly due to being overweight. More than 18 million Americans suffer from this sleep disorder, which causes your airway to collapse during sleep when the muscles in the back of the throat fail to keep the airway open. If you're among those millions, then each night your breathing essentially gets cut off multiple times, and so does that restful sleep. Your sleep becomes fragmented and your blood is not as oxygenated as it should be. Untreated sufferers of sleep apnea never feel fully rested, and this can result in chronic sleep deprivation that raises your risk for a slew of health conditions, from hypertension and heart disease to mood and memory problems.

Symptoms of Sleep Apnea

- You snore.
- You wake up with a headache.
- You're moody most days.
- You're tired to the point of falling asleep during the day.
- You have constant congestion.
- Someone has seen or heard you stop breathing in the middle of the night for brief periods.

Weight and sleep apnea have a strong relationship. The more you weigh—and, specifically, the larger the circumference of your neck—the higher your risk for sleep apnea. Several treatments are available for this condition, one of which is simply losing weight.

For more information about sleep apnea and other sleep-related disorders, visit the National Sleep Foundation at www.sleepfoundation.org.

Another way to ensure healthy sleep is to start keeping records when you have a restless night's sleep. The answer is probably right there somewhere for you to spot where you could be going wrong in your quest for a good night's sleep. There's always a reason why things such as this happen to the body. See if you can keep a record of sleep for a month, alongside a track of what activities you do during the day and when. You can also add your eating and drinking habits to enhance this overall picture. Start to see the triggers of your poor sleep and then focus on avoiding them. Is it too much caffeine? Heated conversations at dinner? Late-night eating, bill paying, and e-mailing? As you mine your data, experiment with new strategies around bedtime. Most people don't keep good records, especially on themselves, but you'd be surprised by how much you can sleuth and interpret yourself if you pay attention.

Remember, sleep is just one activity in the chain of events you undergo each day that contribute or take away from your health. What you do during the day will undoubtedly affect your sleep at night. As I've said throughout, regularity 24-7 is the goal. Far too often we learn to suppress our body's preferred schedule to meet goals that might satisfy other areas of our lives but shift us further from health. Life needn't be monotonous and boring, but when it's rhythmic and imbued with predictability, the body responds positively. If it didn't, then Olympic and professional athletes wouldn't spend so much of their training time regulating their bodies through rigid schedules.

You Can Never Start Too Early

The benefits of adequate sleep extend far beyond what's been documented on adults. When it comes to teaching good sleep hygiene, parents can never start too early. One new study that explored the sleep habits of preschoolers found that bedtime rituals and rules play a unique role in the development of four-year-olds.

It appears that early learning and brain development can be impacted by the bedtime practices that parents keep. When California researchers analyzed a federal survey of some eight thousand families in which parents were asked a slew of questions about bedtime (e.g., "What time does your child go to bed?" and "Do you as parents have a rule about bedtime?"), they surprisingly found that having a rule about bedtime was associated with higher scores on language and math skills. In addition to studying the survey, the researchers followed up with home visits, during which they conducted one-on-one assessments to measure math and language skills.

Children of parents who reported having a rule about bedtime scored about 6 percentage points higher on an assessment of their vocabulary compared with children whose parents did not report a rule about bedtime. They scored 7 percent higher on assessments of early math skills. The differences between the children with rules and those whose bedtime customs were less rigid were significant enough to merit attention. Studies done on teenagers and college students have further confirmed the benefits of regular, restful sleep on performance and test scores.

For parents with children who don't sleep well, some of the studies have been downright scary. In 2010, a study of 392 boys and girls found that those who had trouble sleeping at twelve to fourteen years old were more than two times as likely to have suicidal thoughts at ages fifteen to seventeen as those who didn't have sleep problems at the younger age. A study of 1,037 children revealed that 46 percent of those who were considered to have a persistent sleep difficulty at age nine had an anxiety disorder at age twenty-one or twenty-six. By comparison, of the children who didn't have sleep problems at age nine, 33 percent had an anxiety disorder as young adults.

We don't know why poor sleep in childhood increases the risk of anxiety disorders and depression, but clearly grown-up problems can start in childhood, and some may start at bedtime. It could be that sleep problems lead to changes in the brain, which could, in turn, contribute to the psychiatric illnesses. Anxiety disorders and depression are the most common mental illnesses: 28.8 percent of the general population will be diagnosed with an anxiety disorder in their lifetime and 20.8 percent will be diagnosed with a mood disorder, according to a 2005 study published in the *Archives of General Psychiatry*. Anxiety disorders emerge early in life: the median age of onset is eleven. Rates of depression spike in adolescence, too. Moreover, those who develop depression at a young age tend to develop a more serious form of the disease, with a higher risk of relapse after treatment.

What's a Good Night?

According to the American Academy of Sleep Medicine, children need to sleep:

Infants: 14 to 15 hours
Toddlers: 12 to 14 hours
Preschoolers: 11 to 13 hours
School-age kids: 10 to 11 hours
Teenagers: 9 to 10 hours

Remember, sleep doesn't discriminate based on age. True, we need more or less sleep at different times in our lives, but sleep is nonetheless vital to our well-being—to oiling and fueling that state of equilibrium in our bodies.

These facts do not bode well for the juvenile insomniac, but the good news is that achieving restful sleep is, as I've already implied, easier than most people think. As with adults, kids need a consistent bedtime and wake time, even on weekends. They also need calming bedtime rituals, which could be as simple as reading, taking a bath, and of course limiting any stimulating technology during the half hour before bedtime. The light from computers and TVs can actually suppress the body's production of melatonin, the hormone that promotes sleep. Video games, television, and Web surfing are stimulating to the brain, so shut these off once the bedtime hour has been reached. Parents can often underestimate the stress that their kids bear, so help them to review happy moments from the day before turning off the lights. If they have any worries, relegate those thoughts to a list for tackling the next day. Lastly, try to avoid sending a kid to bed as punishment or to allow them to stay up late as a reward for good behavior. This delivers a negative message about sleep.

Don't Forget Downtime in Your Waking Hours

Earlier I mentioned how sleep allows us to consolidate our memories and prepare to learn new tasks and facts. In this way, sleep acts like a built-in technology application for our brains, cleaning out old files and prepping us to upload new ones. However, sleep isn't the only "application" we need to achieve a fresh, fit mind. We also need downtime in our waking hours. We need a break from our digital devices—a bona fide disconnect from the external forces of technology so that our internal forces can catch up.

Technologies such as those found in our phones and computers, including handheld conveniences, make the smallest windows of time entertaining and potentially productive. But from regular use of these devices we may suffer from an unanticipated side effect:

when we keep our brains busy with digital input, we could be forfeiting downtime that could allow us to better learn and remember information, or to come up with new ideas. A few cases in point make this very clear, as there's mounting evidence that skipping downtime takes a neurological toll.

At the University of California, San Francisco, scientists found that when rats have a new experience, such as exploring an unfamiliar area, their brains show new patterns of activity. But only when the rats take a break from their exploration do they process those patterns in a way that seems to create a persistent memory of the experience. The researchers suspect that the findings also apply to how we learn as humans. Downtime lets the brain take a breather and go over experiences it's had, solidify them, and turn them into permanent long-term memories. When the brain is constantly stimulated, we could be preventing this learning process.

In 2008 at the University of Michigan, researchers discovered a distinct difference between refreshing and fatiguing the brain. Their study found that people learned significantly better after a walk in nature than after a walk in a dense urban environment, suggesting that processing a barrage of information tires the brain. So even though people feel entertained, even relaxed, when they multitask by passing a moment while in line at the supermarket watching a quick video clip or checking e-mail on their phones, they might be taxing their brains in ways we are unable to measure fully.

The moral of the story is that we all need to call a time-out, and more often than we'd probably wish given the volume of distractions we increasingly encounter. The mobile software developers aren't going to quit, and they will find ever-more ways to compete for your time and satisfy your urge to fill up every minute (and in some cases, seconds) with stimulating activities. After all, pretty much everyone with a modern cell phone knows the ongoing pressures to stay connected. How much cortisol do we release when we face a barrage of unanswered e-mails first thing in the morning?

The consequences of being a multitasking digital demon have already been detailed by others, but I'd like to highlight a few choice observations made recently as they pertain to our culture of obsessive hyperconnectivity. At Stanford, for instance, researchers showed that heavy multimedia users have trouble filtering out irrelevant information, as well as focusing tasks. This then starts to take a toll on productivity. Other research says that heavy video-game playing may release dopamine, which is thought to be involved with addictive behaviors. Though we're only just beginning to study the effects of modern life on our brains, it helps to keep in mind that the brain effectively processes only one stream of information at a time. Trying to process multiple streams of information at one time is akin to being at a dinner party where you're hearing several conversations going on at the same time: you can't possibly tune in to all of them. When you apply that concept to a work environment in which you're multitasking—trying to juggle multiple conversations at once, or answering e-mails while talking on the phone—your brain is constantly switching gears. As you move from one task to the next quickly, and then back again, your brain becomes less effective.

In 2010, newspaper reporter Matthew Richtel won the Pulitzer Prize for National Reporting for his article series "Driven to Distraction," which ran in the *New York Times*. The articles focused on the troubling collision of twentieth- and twenty-first-century technologies—specifically driving and multitasking. His synthesis and overview of the research is quite stunning. Some of his conclusions are enough to startle any parent: heavy technology use may fundamentally alter the frontal lobe during childhood. In addition, Richtel covers how addictive behavior can lead to poor decision making and how the highly impressionable young brain is rewired when it is constantly inundated with new information.

In my opinion, one of the best takeaways from Richtel's work is his idea for utilizing this research to make better decisions in our own lives. According to him, we should think of technology in the same way that we think about food. Just as food nourishes us and we need it for life, so, too, do we need technology. You cannot survive without these communication tools; the productivity tools they allow are essential. "And yet," Richtel says, "food has pros and cons to it. We know that some food is junk food and some food is healthy. And we know that if we overeat, it causes problems. Similarly, after 20 years of glorifying technology as if all computers were good and all use of it was good, science is beginning to embrace the idea that some technology is Twinkies and some technology is Brussels sprouts."

And what about the inundation of data? It's been estimated that 25 percent of our workdays are spent immersed in information overload, and indeed, some of that information is Twinkies and some is Brussels sprouts. So not only do we lack true downtime, but we also miss true thinking time, which can help us separate the wheat from the chaff. As we habitually use technology (and, let's admit, demand immediacy) in both retrieving information and tendering our responses, we scatter our attention. I love how Daniel Patrick Forrester, author of *Consider: Harnessing the Power of Reflective Thinking in Your Organization*, puts it in talking about the myth of multitasking. He writes, "Many of us depend on multitasking as the only way to get everything done. However . . . you do an injustice to everything and everyone you're splitting time between. We're sequential beings, not simultaneous. One thing at a time: it's been around as a basic principle since the dawn of time!"

Consider Getting a Dog

Can't stick to a routine? Planning on getting regular sleep and scheduling routine downtime has the overall effect of forcing set patterns that foster health. For those of you who find it extremely challenging to do so, then you might want to consider getting a dog to help out. It's long been anecdotally known that dog owners are often the happiest, most upbeat people. But it's not all about the companionship of having a pooch to love and care for—owning a dog demands that a person maintain a relatively constant and reliable timetable, tending to the animal's ritualistic feedings, walks, and naps. This often means sticking to a regular schedule. It also helps that walking a dog forces its owner to move, to engage in at least some physical exercise, even if Fido isn't a feisty greyhound looking for a run. The combination of this regularity of schedule and forced exercise, however strenuous, is a dynamic duo. Being outside in nature with dogs also offers the benefits of downtime, as walking dogs demands that the owners vacate their computer desks and cease multitasking, besides scooping up poop and talking on their cell phones at the same time.

You might be wondering if these benefits also extend to parents of real people, not dogs. The tendency here is to automatically assume that parents would fall into similar patterns with their children, who need constant and relatively consistent attention around sleeping and eating habits. While it's true that parents fall into patterns with their children, kids' needs and demands can change, especially on a whim, and this makes for erratic schedules at times. Dogs lead more predictable and simple lives. Growing, developing children with a much higher level of brain activity and learning capacity require more from us. However, they still need regular routines in their lives as much as we do for good health.

Health Rule

Keep a strict, predictable schedule 365 days a year that has you eating, sleeping, and exercising at about the same times day in and day out. Avoid napping unless you nap every single day at the same time. Respect regularity. Schedule downtime. Share this knowledge with your children.

PART III

The Future You

The saddest aspect of life right now is that science gathers
knowledge faster than society gathers wisdom.

—*Isaac Asimov,* Isaac Asimov's Book of Science
and Nature Quotations, *1988*

There's a slogan about the last century being the century of
the physical sciences and the twenty-first century being the
century of the biological sciences. I respectfully disagree and
believe that we are entering a century of the convergence and unity
of all sciences. As I've said before, the marriage of technology and
medicine will be one of history's most fruitful unions.

Life may well be a marathon, which I stated in chapter 10, but we
each need to run it as if we're playing a game of chess. You'll move
one piece at a time and change the game as you go. Science may
never cure the condition or disease that may strike you, and you may

not be able to entirely avoid it for whatever reason. But you can most definitely reduce how much it affects you and change how you treat yourself through its progression. Cancer might one day become a chronic disease much like diabetes. We'll learn to control and manage it better. As with diseases such as diabetes, one of the ways we'll manage it is by knowing its biology, and the way we know this is by monitoring the way your body responds to a drug. All the molecular tests in the world are far less important and meaningful than your body's response to a drug. We have to learn from every action we take, as we do during a chess game, and chart every reaction to our action. In strategizing against a wily opponent such as cancer, we have to make a move, think ahead, and watch what the enemy does.

Health Rule

Don't think too much about where you'll be healthwise in ten years. Just focus on the present year. That's it, because medical technology changes too fast. You don't know what's going to happen in the future. Everything is probabilistic when you think about it—not deterministic. Do not rely on a textbook to tell you about something that might happen in ten years. Medicine is so dynamic and ever-changing, you should instead be attached to that hope. Some people live to the day they die; others die the day they are diagnosed. But one of the most important things to remember here is studies have proven that people live longer when they have an optimistic outlook.

My goal as a doctor is to keep people healthy for ten years. By the time we reach that ten-year mark, I firmly believe that we'll have discovered some other way to better your health. We'll have new therapies, new treatments, and new roads to take. If you don't respond well to a drug or if you begin to lose hope that you'll survive an illness looming in your distant future, such as Alzheimer's disease, don't waste too much time worrying; be optimistic and help yourself to be more relaxed by thinking and strategizing in ten-year increments.

In the same spirit as this ten-year plan, I also want to propose that you follow what I call the one-year rule. Every year, go through your list of drugs with your doctor and see if you can knock a few off. Experiment with going off them to see if you still need them all. Obviously, you may be taking a drug that your doctor will not advise you modify or stop. But this exercise can be informative. See if you still have that joint problem. See if you still have high blood pressure. Keep in mind that the technology of drugs changes, too. If you've been on the same drug, perhaps you should be asking, is it still right for you? It helps to also do the same for any supplements and over-the-counter medications that you take regularly. I watch so many patients come in with a laundry list of bottles, which sit in their medicine cabinets or kitchen cupboards, and like brushing their teeth or taking out the trash, they pop their pills and down their elixirs—practically unconsciously. I'd like to see people give much greater consideration to the drugs they're taking and determine exactly what benefits these hold for their bodies.

One of the more important takeaways of this book, which I've (hopefully) been driving home since the beginning, is that I want you to appreciate the dynamism of the body. It's constantly changing—second after second with each breath you take and year after year as you age. All of us make slight shifts in our lives routinely even when we don't realize it, and this can be as subtle as banking more hours of sleep, biking to work, and buying 1 percent fat milk instead of 2 percent. Those slights shifts add up. So while you may think that your body needs a constant supply of certain drugs, think again. Health is a constantly moving target. Just as you check yourself in the mirror before stepping out the door in the morning, you would do well to check your medicine cabinets at least once a year.

As you're about to learn in this last part, you would also do well to keep abreast of emerging technologies and take advantage of them when they are available to you. The ten-year rule exists because I have no doubt that we'll be in a totally different place ten years from now. The technologies that are emerging thanks to revolutionary advancements being made in the digital and computational arena are truly astounding and will propel my field of medicine to unprecedented heights.

12

High-Tech Health

How Virtual Reality and Knowledge from the
Video Game World May One Day Save Our Lives

When I picture what it will be like for my two kids to take care of themselves and stay in good health as independent adults further down the road, I imagine that they will be able to walk into their doctor's office and have their finger pricked to leave a small sample of blood on a biochip, which will be assessed in a way that allows them to work with their primary physician to create a personalized plan of action attuned to their unique physiological needs. This type of treatment isn't far from what was featured in the 1997 movie *Gattaca* (made up of the letters from the four bases in human DNA—adenine, cytosine, guanine, and thymine). In that movie, a genetically inferior man, played by Ethan Hawke, assumes the identity of a superior one to pursue his lifelong dream of space travel. He learns to deceive DNA and urine-sample testing, but the plot thickens the closer he gets to liftoff. I don't believe that our culture will ever live the way it does in some of these futuristic sci-fi movies where society analyzes people's DNA and determines whether they measure up to certain standards. Much to the contrary, I see a world where those who take advantage of new technologies will reap enormous benefits in terms of their health and ability to gain control of their well-being in unfathomable ways.

For my children and, later, grandchildren, the information gleaned by the examination of their blood will inform their health strategy, which will entail a combination of preventive measures and perhaps some therapies for treating identified ailments or signs of "unhealthiness." By that I mean indicators that the body has shifted away from a healthy state somewhere in its complex network. This can be any number of things or symptoms, from imbalances in blood-sugar control (i.e., a risk factor for diabetes) to uncontrolled cell growth, which could signal cancer. What is equally exciting is that their sample, and its related annotation, will add to a universal database, increasing the utility of this database daily.

In this scenario, blood won't be the only fluid that we will be able to examine for clues to health and the absence of health. We'll probably be able to observe what's happening in tears, saliva, urine, lymphatic fluid, spinal fluid, and so on. But blood does have some key advantages. It's wonderful that we all have a collecting system built into our bodies that goes around and touches every place in our body and collects fluids. Blood is convenient for diagnostics; it's relatively easy to extract, and because it delivers nutrients and gets rid of waste, it's pretty much involved in anything dramatic that's happening in the body. It's a great starting point for measuring the state of the body.

It's amazing that a doctor today looks at things on the outside of you, takes your temperature, tells you to hop on a scale, maybe checks a few specific ingredients in your blood such as sodium and white blood cell count, and decides what you should do. This partly explains why we've gravitated toward diagnostic treatment medicine rather than active preventive medicine. With limited knowledge, diagnostic medicine makes sense. If we don't know what we're trying to prevent or how best to go about doing that, then we have to wait for an obvious symptom to emerge in order to take action. At that point, we're usually treating a disease that has had ample opportunity to progress. A much better, more effective approach would be to base our personal care on known parameters—parameters that can be measured. Thankfully, technologies are finally emerging for us to measure and define these parameters.

Once we had the ability to play with genes, everyone thought, "This will be great, we'll delete gene X or Y and see what breaks." Probably the biggest surprise was that when you turn off or "knock out" a gene in a model system such as a mouse, at least half the time nothing seems to break. One broken gene doesn't result in a catastrophe because something else in the system probably takes up the slack. Somewhere in the system there has to be a redundancy that can be a lifesaver.

Engineers know about the value of redundancy. Take an airplane, for instance, which cannot fail due to a single glitch in the system. If airplanes could fall from the sky following one malfunction, no one would dare step on a plane. The airline industry couldn't persuade people to risk their lives in the face of such a strong and realistic possibility. We know how faulty humans can be, so the thought of a maintenance-crew member forgetting to screw a bolt in correctly or neglecting to notice a chip in the wing is all too vivid. And it could happen in an instant. Which is why airplanes are somewhat immune to malfunctions due to improper maintenance; they have built-in redundancies to avert such fates. Only when several malfunctions happen in sequence or, God forbid, all at once do problems arise. Of course, if the pilot is ill-trained in handling an escalating dilemma, then we've got the possibility of human error to add to this potential catastrophe (though some planes are even smarter than that with automated systems that can take over the controls to avoid human error). So the implication is clear: redundancies are a good thing. They keep people alive, not just in capsules zooming at thirty thousand feet aboveground, but also at the molecular level—within our bodies, where at least one hundred thousand chemical reactions occur in the brain every second.

Interestingly, evolved systems such as the human body have adapted and developed over time to be robust and redundant. When you think about it, robustness is a form of information hiding. You don't necessarily know when your body loses a critical ingredient because it has a backup plan. Another way to understand this is to consider that your body responds the same under many different circumstances, and with some of its parts broken or faltering once in a while. Your body gets good at concealing the information related to its inner workings. To make something robust is to mask the information at the level of the symptoms, which is the level where your doctor is examining you.

A great example of this in my world is with the BRCA1 gene, which you'll recall is a gene responsible for repairing DNA. Women who inherit a defect on this gene are at much higher risk for experiencing an aggressive form of breast cancer. Even though breast cells are dividing all the time, cancer doesn't occur because DNA repairs are happening under the radar all the time as well. Breast cancer happens down the road for someone with the BRCA1 defect because of an accumulation of problems in the DNA for which the body can no longer compensate. The DNA repair shop is overloaded and can no longer handle the influx of problems. This helps explain why many cancer patients don't have a lot of symptoms in the early stages—the defects haven't reach a point yet where symptoms become evident, and why many patients with BRCA mutations don't develop cancer until later in life.

Your body has evolved to make its systems opaque about what's going on inside. But the body is not only sneaky, it's also quite crafty. For the most part, it fixes itself when it's sick or cancering, but if you can help it at all—tilt it in the right direction—we know that the body has a tremendous capacity to heal.

Ditching the Diagnosis Paradigm

The switch from today's approach of diagnose $\rightarrow$ categorize $\rightarrow$ treat according to established methods, to a much more dynamic, simulated model that is based on personal factors, will have a profound effect on how people take care of themselves and even *think* of themselves. Once we're able to measure several variables that define the true "state" of the body through technologies such as proteomics, we'll be able to realize the promise of personalized medicine. With the comprehensive view that proteomics can give us, we can start to manipulate that picture—and create a picture of health.

As doctors, we'll be able to design personal protocols that serve multiple purposes for individuals. These won't be static protocols. They will be as dynamic as the changes in the state of your body. You'll replan your protocol every time you visit your doctor and he or she remeasures your system. The goals in my industry will also shift. I won't give you a drug to lower your cholesterol; I'll treat you to a non-cardiac-event state. Similarly, I won't treat you to shrink your cancer by 50 percent; I'll treat you to a healthy state whereby the cancer's growth is under control. That's a very different way of approaching medical care and looking at health. The most instrumental weapon of all will no doubt be the products that we will develop to do all this tweaking and early intervening before illness sets up camp in your body.

It should be noted here that much of the system that comprises our healthy body actually doesn't have human DNA at all. It has some other microbial DNA, and we probably are a complicated ecosystem of different types of our own cells and lots of nonhuman microbial cells. In addition to bacterial DNA in our digestive tracts, we are each filled with fungal and viral microbes as well that assist in digestion and participate in our immune response. We have more of these microbes living in our intestinal tract (about 500 trillion or three pounds' worth) than we have cells in our body (only about 80 trillion). As you already read in chapter 8, our microbiome—the totality of microbes, their genetic elements (genomes), and their interactions within us—has a lot to do with our health. It comprises the heart of our immunity and can have a say in functions as diverse as which hormones are rushing through your blood to whether you will likely battle obesity and live with a higher-than-average risk for certain types of cancer. The point is, once we start looking at the whole proteome, we'll actually be looking at the conversation of *all* of those cells—not just the human cells.

So, yes, some of those stripes and dots that showed up in the picture on page 113 correlate to a particular human protein. But, some of those stripes or dots are currently "undefined": we don't know if they might be produced by some combination of other proteins, or if they reflect some other organism's protein that's enjoying the ride in our warm body. That's another of the beauties of proteomics: we can see everything, whether it's human or not, and really begin to draw conclusions.

What you're ultimately trying to do is guide your body back to a healthy state, which here means back to a sort of homeostasis, or a place where you're not misfiring neurotransmitters, you're not experiencing a miscue in your metabolism, you're not harboring a colony of bacteria that puts you at risk for certain ailments, you're not suffering from a blip in your immune system or any system for that matter, and you're certainly not cancering uncontrollably. That's really all that health is, a state of being whereby your system allows you to function on all cylinders and enjoy a high quality of life. This last part of the definition obviously differentiates us from the health of a computer network. In this steady state, the body knows what's going to happen next, its redundancies are working to make up for any minor glitches, and it's on even keel, for the most part. Remember, the body loves predictability. If you can ensure that predictability, say by reducing its load of stress so it can function well, then you stand a greater chance at fostering a healthy state.

The movie *Gattaca* might have left a few people wondering how close we are to manipulating genes to the point we can "transform" ourselves to new human beings capable of extraordinary feats and ultrahuman health. While we may be far from turning ourselves into superheroes that can leap tall buildings in a single bound and have X-ray vision, I do believe that the breakthroughs happening every day, step by step in cutting-edge labs around the world working with genes, proteins, microbes, etc., will change medicine as we know it in our lifetimes. It will amount to a big leap from the day a magazine cover stopped me in my tracks.

A Virtual Reality

For someone such as me who has devoted his life to studying and treating cancer, you can imagine the sucker punch I felt when I walked past my hospital's gift shop and saw the cover of *Fortune* magazine proclaiming "Why We're Losing the War on Cancer." It seemed to be pointing a finger at me telling me how terribly I'd been doing my job. Cancer care has been much criticized over the last several decades, and clearly this article was trying to rip apart my field some more. But, despite my initial reaction, I did and do believe that this kind of criticism is desperately needed, and I am inspired by the challenge to fix what's broken. As I've been advocating throughout this book, if we start to understand that diseases, including cancer, are not just molecular defects, then we'll get to new ways of treating them.

When you consider all the variables to an illness such as cancer, and even if you don't know what all those variables are, you have to understand the data inputs. To understand what I'm getting at, consider what would happen if I measured your temperature over thirty days to arrive at an average. Let's say that your average turned out to be a normal of 98.7 degrees Fahrenheit. I would say great. But if during one of those days your temperature spiked to 102 for six hours, and you took Tylenol and got better, I could have totally missed that spike. This illustrates one of the fundamental problems in medicine: you and I visit our doctor once a year, if that. That single visit allows our physicians to obtain a static measurement of a few data points, such as our temperature, blood pressure, weight, and so on. But your doctor has no way of knowing about all the fluctuations in between visits and how much those data points changed.

As I mentioned earlier, for several months I used a device that told me how many calories I burned each day. This eye-opening experiment showed me what I would certainly have missed had I just calculated my average calorie expenditure by measuring at random points in a twenty-four-hour period. This device mapped all of my activity throughout that twenty-four-hour period and told me that for three hours every day I'm sitting at my desk not moving at all. As we've already seen, being sedentary like that can have tremendous repercussions biologically—basically this upped my risk for a multitude of diseases.

So, if you think of any disease as a system, there's an input and an output and a state in the middle.

The "state" is really just the person as a patient. It's you or me. The input includes factors such as our environment, diet, treatments, and sometimes our genetic mutations. The output includes our symptoms. Do we have pain? Is our condition worsening? Do we feel bloated, etc.? What doctors do is change an input; they give aggressive chemotherapy, for instance, and then they ask, did our output get better? Did our pain improve, etc.? Did our condition get better?

Part of my current quest to improve cancer treatment, which will hopefully inform treatments across the board for a spectrum of maladies, is to bring all this new technology that I've been describing into the virtual world. In 2009 I was part of a team, together with Danny Hillis and Parag Mallick, that put together a proposal for the National Cancer Institute that called for a Physical Sciences in Oncology Center. Our center, which was funded to a tune of $16.2 million by the NCI, has solicited teams from seven leading institutions to develop multiple data sources and dimensions about cancer to allow others to build a "virtual tumor." The data sources for achieving this virtual tumor are as diverse as single-cell sequencing to the "pokability" of the individual cancer cell. When I say "pokability," I mean exactly that: the ability to physically poke a cell with a tiny little instrument the way you would poke someone's shoulder with your finger to get their attention. This may sound like an exceedingly unscientific way to evaluate a cell, but it's actually one of the most sensitive tests we have to study a cell's condition. It's also an effective technique for determining how it responds. A cell's "stiffness" reflects all the underlying biology of that cell and its environment.

Based on all of this information, we can model a cancer and its interactions with the host and develop new and hopefully better strategies to control the cancer. The key to being able to do this is to build a multiscale model, including the cancer cell, the tumor, the organ, and the body. We can start to play with the virtual tumor like a video game and see what happens. What if I mutated this gene? What if I changed the system here? It's hard to believe that we don't perform these kinds of experiments yet. We normally just throw a drug into a patient and then see what happens. But the technology hasn't been mature enough to conduct such an experiment. Until now.

If all this still feels to you a bit like science fiction worthy of a movie starring Ethan Hawke and Uma Thurman, let's briefly turn to one of the most celebrated spectator sports today, which, oddly enough, owes a lot of its drama and interaction to complex computer modeling going on behind the scenes.

What Football Coaches Can Teach
Doctors Seeking Better Cures

Tom Landry, the legendary founding coach of the Dallas Cowboys, brought the team from a winless first season to domination of the National Football League in the 1960s and 1970s. I mention him because over his twenty-nine-year career with the Cowboys, Landry used a variety of engineering techniques to help him build the most successful program in NFL history. From quality control to industrial psychology to computer analysis, Landry used the tools of the engineering profession to lead his team to twenty consecutive winning seasons, an NFL record. Landry was the first coach to use a computer. Today, Landry is immortalized in a namesake video game that is based on his game strategies.

Making use of complex computer modeling in medicine based on how video games work is not as fanciful and abstract as you might think. After all, if it can win Super Bowls, why not wars on disease? If Landry could change the future of football with his computing skills, then why can't today's scientists adopt such similarly minded skills and apply them to the future of medicine? Most of us don't think about how something as playful as video games function, but they are brilliant in their strategy and sophisticated in their craftiness. Based on a set of rules, video games take in an enormous amount of data and match it to certain outcomes in different scenarios. If your virtual character is shot in the head, for example, you die. If you run toward somebody, he steps backward in this virtual world. Every time you play the game, you're testing out rules that have already been built into the system.

In the parallel universe of the real world where we've got opposing teams such as cancer, autoimmune and neurodegenerative diseases, wouldn't it be nice if we could have all the input data for a certain affliction and play with a virtual version to see what happens? We could, theoretically, turn a gene on and see what happens to a cancerous tumor. Much in the way kids spend hours figuring out clever ways to shoot a bad guy in a video game, I want researchers to spend their days figuring out how to kill a cancer cell. Or how we can deliver chemotherapy without side effects. I know that we can do that if we create a reliable cancer gaming system. Just as Landry could create a computer model based on the statistics-rich history of the NFL, we can start to do the same in the world of medicine. We'll take statistics from the history of cancer, for example, and all that we know about cancer to date, and start to build the model that will enable us to claim victory in a game we all want to win.

Over the next decade doctors will start to approach diseases more like weather forecasters than biologists. Thirty years ago we couldn't predict the weather all that precisely. But then we developed climate models to predict patterns, and today we can provide ten-day forecasts that are pretty darn accurate. Weather forecasting went from being reliant on a farmers' almanac that was published once a year, and which gave general, vague notions of what people could expect based on seasons, to a high-tech, real-time industry that has the added benefit of saving lives. This technology is improving year by year with more advanced computer modeling—examining the shape of the clouds, temperature changes, moisture, etc. We can predict hurricanes, blizzards, tornadoes, and monsoons, for instance, and better prepare for them. But we can't right now do the same in my field because not enough information has been collected and organized for such an ambitious endeavor. We now need this massive collection of data more than anything else. Just as a computer can study the shape of a cloud and predict a weather pattern, so, too, should a computer be able to study the shape of a tumor and say something about the cancer's rate of growth, blood supply, nutrients, and anatomical location, among other things.

Another way to look at the power of this kind of technology is to consider what marketers do when they test out new shelving techniques on sales figures. They constantly test out new strategies to garner more sales: *When I place the product at eye level, do sales go up? What about here? Where is the ideal spot to display my product to attract more customers?* Likewise, what is the ideal set of conditions for the body to maximize health? As a patient, you'll be able to ask, what happens when I take drug X or therapy Y? How can I optimize my system with the foods I eat, the activities I engage in, and the sports I play? Equally, which things should I avoid or limit?

Other questions will also be part of this ongoing negotiation, for you'll have to consider what you want your body to do for you. You'll have to determine what your metrics should be to arrive at the body you want. A bodybuilder, for instance, will have a different set of metrics from a concert pianist. A corporate executive whose blood pressure surges every afternoon like clockwork will focus his efforts on controlling that metric, just as the insomniac's goal will be to achieve restful sleep nine times out of ten. So not only will people's individual metrics vary, but how they prioritize their metrics will also follow unique patterns. Still, despite these variations, there will be one huge commonality: a collective spirit for sharing, which will be critical to the success of this new approach to health.

Health Rule

Always be thinking in terms of your body's system. It has inputs and outputs. Collect data regarding yourself and store it in an easily accessible place, as your doctor will need to analyze this to make educated interpretations of the health of your system. Your set of information, or metrics, will be unique to you—allowing you to custom-tailor your health plan to your needs. It's one size fits *you, not all.*

13

The Give-and-Take

*How Sharing Our Medical Information
Can Make Us Live Longer and Better*

I am routinely dazzled by stories that confirm what I've long
thought to be true. In the fall of 2008, a most remarkable thing
happened: a search engine predicted a flu outbreak three weeks
before the Centers for Disease Control. But this didn't surprise me,
for I knew that search-engine technology would eventually outpace
old-fashioned methods of tracking illness and disease. But I was a
bit amazed by the transformational impact of this event—and how it
could revolutionize a lot in medicine far from issues of public health.

Each week, millions of people around the world search for health
information online. As you might expect, more flu-related searches
occur during the winter, more allergy-related searches in the spring,
and more sunburn-related searches over the summer. You can
explore all of these phenomena using Google Insights for Search,
which allows you to compare search volume patterns across specific

regions, categories, time frames, and properties. For example, you can see where people are searching for the word *merlot* or *cabernet*. Likewise, you can narrow your search to a geographic location and see what *soccer in Brazil*, for instance, turns up. This kind of tool can help businesses find customers, anticipate demand for products or services, and track general trends. But can search-query trends provide the basis for an accurate, reliable model of real-world phenomena?

That is the question that Larry Brilliant, a champion epidemiologist, technologist, and one of the leaders of the successful World Health Organization smallpox-eradication program, wanted to answer a few years ago. At the time, he was director of Google's philanthropic arm, Google.org, and joined forces with other curious colleagues to perform a little experiment. Actually, it turned out to be a big experiment spanning the globe and peeking into pockets of communities where people were typing words such *fever, chill*, and *flu* into their computers at unusual rates. Indeed, Brilliant found a close relationship between how many people search for flu-related topics and how many people actually have flu symptoms. Of course, not every person who searches for *flu* is actually sick, but a pattern emerges when all the flu-related search queries are added together, a technique called aggregated search data. Brilliant's team compared their query counts with traditional flu surveillance systems, such as those used by the CDC, and found that many search queries tend to be popular exactly when flu season is happening and where the outbreaks are—all over the world. By counting how often they saw these search queries, they could estimate how much flu was circulating in different countries and regions around the world. Thus Google Flu Trends was born, and their results were published in the journal *Nature*. (You can download the Google Flu Trends estimates for weekly influenza activity around the world at http://www .google.org/flutrends.)

Before you dwell on issues of privacy, it should be duly noted that

Google Flu Trends can never be used to identify individual users because it relies on anonymous, aggregated counts of how often certain search queries occur each week. It relies on millions of search queries issued to Google over time, and the patterns it observes in the data are only meaningful across large populations of Google search users.

Imagine, for a moment, the power of this technology. Seasonal influenza epidemics are a major public health concern, causing tens of millions of respiratory illnesses and 250,000 to 500,000 deaths worldwide each year. In addition to seasonal influenza, a new strain of influenza virus against which no previous immunity exists and that is transmissible human-to-human could result in a pandemic with millions of fatalities. The swine flu scare that occurred in 2009 will someday be dwarfed by a real epidemic that will spread rapidly through virgin immune systems and kill millions in its path (as happened, for example, in the flu pandemic of 1918, when an estimated 50 million to 100 million people died).

Early detection of disease activity, however, when followed by a rapid response, can reduce the impact of both seasonal and pandemic influenza. Clearly, one way to improve early detection is to monitor health-seeking behavior as Google.org did, which luckily has access to millions of people around the world each day in real time. Why bother with estimates from aggregated search queries? Traditional flu surveillance is important, but most health agencies focus on a single country or region and only update their estimates once per week at most. That Google Flu Trends can monitor trends in near real time makes it an exquisitely powerful tool. I encourage you to check out the animated video on the website, which clearly demonstrates the speed with which Google predicted flu outbreaks in the mid-Atlantic region of the United States in the winter of 2008. The CDC's data lagged a few weeks behind Google. Weeks, when it comes to spotting increases in flu, can mean the difference between life and death for those who don't see the disaster coming.

The Google trending phenomenon brings up another good point: technologies such as those behind Google's masterful search engine that can take data sets with known outcomes and organize them can and should be employed by medicine. My hope is that with new applications that make genomics and now proteomics a valuable area of rapid study, we can start to collect information in a manner that will return ever-more data—data that we can use to further understand our individual systems. Yes, this means sharing your "system" with the world for someone else to benefit. Before you contemplate the privacy debate and attempt to throw tomatoes, let me clarify. This isn't about labeling you with certain diseases and chronic conditions and then revealing your name and label online for the world to see. This is about democratizing our health data in a way that makes it accessible and usable to researchers who can study all this information and find new solutions. I have little concern about writing a check or paying a credit card online with the

> The Internet transmits an enormous amount of health-care-related information, the majority of it being medical images. Zero percent of those images are organized in any useful manner to be helpful in enhancing your health or even saving your life. Moreover, there is no standard terminology for medical terms. For example, you call it a broken leg and I call it a fractured leg. Current search engine technology treats these as two different things.

click of a mouse, but would I be worried about anonymously giving someone such as Google my cholesterol level? Not in the least. If doing so would allow me to better understand how I can control my cholesterol and support my healthy goal state, then why not? I'd love for my genomic and proteomic data to be anonymously donated to technologies like that so it can mine my information and tell me something I don't know. A significant amount of all traffic on the Internet is medical related. But none of it is organized in any useful fashion. We're generating staggering amounts of data daily, but it's going nowhere to return any rewards to us later and perhaps save our lives.

All of us need to participate in a global melting pot of health data. It's part of what I call the give-and-take. You and I will have an active role in building this global virtual health model that can change the course of not just our health, but the health of our children, our neighbors, and the world at large. Google successfully created a hash table for the Internet, and now we need to create our own hash table of the human body. In the end, American health will be saved by its most important virtue: an informed and willing patient.

A New Kind of Health-Care Reform

I'm not going to step far into this murky subject other than to say that we, as a human race—not as politicking individuals with agendas and opinions—will owe much of the reform we need in health care to how we each choose to participate in this global vision of health. I mean that seriously: much of the current banter is about health-care finance reform. But we need health-care reform at a much more basic and fundamental level before we can get to the financial end of it. When I use that term *health care*, I'm referring to how I, you, and everyone else goes about caring for their health and exchanging health information.

As more and more people willingly, anonymously add their health data to a growing database, the information will gather strength and momentum. It will demand to be organized and mined. The key will be in transforming all this information into real knowledge, which will require the creation of a hierarchy—similar to what Google does when it returns a hierarchy of outcomes following your input of search terms. Google's programs return search outcomes that match your query and are ordered from top to bottom based on what you most likely care about from most to least. Imagine that kind of personalized data returned to you about your health and how you can make the most use of it.

Obviously we're not yet at a point where you can benefit from this kind of technology. But what I'm offering is more than a proposition because I do believe we'll get there, and personalized medicine will involve technologies that reflect an amalgam of all the sciences, including computer engineering.

To propel this movement forward, I believe that we'll need to create incentives.

The Power of Incentives

It's been proven again and again that the human spirit runs on incentives. We are a goal-driven society, especially in America, where we are inspired largely by the promise of independence, free will, prosperity, and certain personal rights that we take seriously. Without goals and incentives, most of us lack the motivation to do anything. It's hard to lift ourselves out of bed unless we have a job to go to that pays the bills and feeds our families. Some of us refuse to change our habit of working a hundred hours a week unless our spouse threatens to leave us. We fail to eat well most of the time unless the fear of ill health and the desire to lose weight are great enough to make us choose quinoa over country-fried steak. As some of my colleagues like to point out, there's no better cure for smoking than cancer or emphysema.

You may have noticed in our culture recently an outcropping of our deep-seated need for personal freedom coupled with the demand for information to make good decisions in our free lives. It's called collaboration—a sharing of knowledge, creativity, skills, and whatever should be exchanged in pursuit of progress and preservation of personal freedom. Collaboration has taken the business world by storm in the past decade, yielding new advancements and technologies aplenty. Some would argue that we owe much of the digital improvements that we enjoy today to this constant dialogue between consumers and businesses that helps us create what we want and eventually find invaluable. The rise in consumerism has arguably catapulted our society to a place where cocreation and collaboration reign supreme. More recently, we witnessed what happens when technology and collaboration are paired together to mobilize peoples and whole countries. It brought down regimes in Tunisia and Egypt and called into question the very concept of what it means for a hold on power to be "ironclad." Power, and particularly the power to change things, resides not in rulers steeped in a long history of authoritarianism, but in a collective force that has power by its sheer numbers and will. There have always been uprisings and changes in leadership in countries, but the time scale for change has radically changed. In weeks, not years, real change was enacted through the collaboration of the people using the tools of social media.

But such collaboration has yet to enter the health world. The heart and soul of collaboration is the absolute opposite of reductionist, ironclad thinking. Earlier I mentioned how I picture my kids as adults dropping a small sample of body fluid off at their doctors' offices from which they will be able to learn what they can do better to improve their health. I don't envision them going to a single room in a building that houses several doctors working in their own vacuums. Quite the contrary, I hope that they have the opportunity to enter a building that houses practicing doctors, laboratory researchers, drug developers, clinics, operating rooms, physical therapists, overnight patients, and so on. I think we'd all get a different sense of health and disease if we could witness simultaneously all the moving parts of the health industry that currently operate as separate entities. Wouldn't it be great if all the players in the health-care field worked together and continually watched what each other was doing daily? I also imagine lots of glass-encased rooms so passersby can peer inside to see the action taking place.

It's absurd that most cancer biologists today have never observed surgery. This is the equivalent of an astrophysicist who has never peered into a telescope. Most cancer biologists think of surgery as having an absolute outcome—you either "get" the cancer or you don't. They neither realize or appreciate the chaos of cancer. We don't know the beginning and the end of cancer, which is why it's so terrifying. We may be justified in fearing cancer for this reason. But where we wrong ourselves is in directing similar fears onto the notion of sharing and collaborating in personal medicine, which must start at the patient level. It must start with you and me.

Sadly, many of us still hold tightly to obsolete fears over loss of privacy and autonomy when it comes to sharing our medical records. Until we democratize our medical data so as to protect each individual's privacy but at the same time to allow us to share critical information that can fuel a new industry of research and innovation, then we might as well stay stuck in the current era of stagnation. The more data we have, the less error. The power to change the course of medicine and the future of our individual health resides not in governments but in our joined efforts.

Twenty years ago we scoffed at the thought of conducting all of our banking and bill-paying online. Fewer than ten years ago many of us would have cringed at the notion of uploading personal photos and snippets of our thoughts to websites such as Facebook and Twitter that can be accessed from all over the world. But now these activities are second nature, and they can be downright empowering. They allow us to connect, to build community, to take control of our lives in ways that we wouldn't otherwise be able to. And they are vehicles through which we can express our personal integrity, sense of self-determination, and sovereignty.

The first time I heard about Michael Dell's Well at Dell program, which helps employees track and manage their health care, I knew he was on to something. In 2004, Dell, the world's largest computer manufacturer, designed Well at Dell to encourage healthy lifestyles and incentivize employees to participate in its health-improvement programs, such as by participating in health surveys, using the on-site fitness centers, and switching over to electronic health records that can manage insurance claims and drug prescriptions. Other companies, including Cisco, have adopted similar programs.*

Dell is revolutionizing the whole concept of corporate wellness. Its program has since been upgraded to capture new information about treatments and test results easily without having to wait for the employee to enter the data manually. Dell's dedication to health care has made it the largest purveyor of health-care information in the country. It doesn't just create computer-based systems to manage its own internal health care, but it builds and maintains systems for other companies to benefit from in their own health-care management. Cisco Systems has a similar-minded health-care facility and means to track its employees' records at its headquarters in San Jose.

I'd be naive to think that programs like this don't stir controversy, but bear with me for a moment. You might squirm at the thought of your employer handling your medical records and telling you about new ways to better your health, but what these companies have done can actually make health care more efficient and allow money to be spent where it needs to be spent—on people like you and me rather than administration. Such a system has built-in mechanisms to maintain the privacy of employees, but the tremendous power of

---

*To clarify, I should emphasize that these programs are not mandatory. Employees choose to opt in and they control all of their own data, including who gets to see what. These programs are not intended to monitor employees' health and lifestyle choices. They are solely intended to help employees keep themselves and their families healthy by offering them services and benefits that they would otherwise not receive. These opportunities ultimately help to improve health and reduce out-of-pocket medical insurance costs for everyone.

these programs allows employees to receive alerts and information customized to their health issues, concerns, goals, and even their test results so that they can make more informed decisions in their health care.

For example, a newly diagnosed diabetic might get information about how to monitor blood sugar and how to care for his or her feet, since diabetics suffer complications ranging from skin changes to circulatory problems that can sometimes lead to amputation. The system can also have its benefits providers use data-mining software to look for patterns in an employee's medical care. Patients with identifiable health conditions or risk factors will then be invited into health-coaching programs. An overweight employee, for instance, who has high blood pressure and prediabetes can participate in a workshop designed to help him learn practical strategies to losing weight and improving his health profile without having to resort to drugs. Put simply, Dell's and Cisco's systems facilitate a means through which employees can gain information relevant to them so that they can stay on top of their total wellness. The ultimate goal for Dell and Cisco is to empower their people to take charge of their preventive medicine. The programs are about giving—not taking away. Programs such as these are not intended to negatively affect people in terms of their insurance coverage or how much they have to pay.

Not surprisingly, companies such as Cisco and Dell that offer some kind of employee-directed, online health-management tool have their critics, most of whom belabor the issues revolving around privacy and Big Brother. After all, few of us want someone else to badger us to drop twenty pounds, join a gym, and buy more fruits and vegetables lest we lose our job. As part of our entitlement to certain freedoms, we don't like having to live by someone else's "house" rules in the workplace. But this is less about the debate over who is boss and who is going to pay for our medical care than it is about achieving the best possible health care that we can. We can't have it both ways: we can't expect our health-care industry to continue to innovate and grow if we continue to hoard our health information. The federal agency that administers Medicare pays for over half of the medical bills in this country, yet it doesn't retrieve, organize, or mine any of that data. I can only imagine how much better the Medicare system could be if all the data that filters through Medicare's office alone were recorded, examined, and analyzed to better public health.

Or, on a smaller scale, just think about what happens when you visit your general practitioner and he finds something that he wants you to check out further with another doctor, who is probably located in another building or part of the city. Let's say your doctor finds a lump in your breast. He orders a mammogram and refers you to this other doctor. Suddenly, you've got three different people in this picture—your GP, the radiologist who will read your mammogram, and the specialist who (hopefully) knows a lot about breasts and will determine which course of treatment, if any, you need.

Then a biopsy follows, so enter the surgeon and pathologist. Maybe there's even another doctor or specialist called in if you ask for a second opinion. By the time you return to your GP weeks later for follow-up, you've been through a crowd of various health-care workers. The data flow between these doctors is negligible, but the data created by each doctor is staggering. You probably don't have a single copy of any of that data on hand, so when you land in the emergency room three days later because you slipped and fell in your driveway, you don't have any of that information to hand over. Your breast biopsy may have nothing to do per se with the injury you sustained in the fall, but lots of other information in your file could probably help the ER doctors take excellent care of you.

I don't want this to sound like a caustic rant or diatribe against people who lead less-than-perfect lifestyles, who are probably the least likely to want to share their medical information. We all have our vices. This is more about incentives than penalties. It's about creating powerful motives that can trump deterrents to healthy living. The underlying message here should be obvious: check out your company's corporate wellness program if it has one. Many large companies today are creating the incentives we need to stay active and to pay attention to our health, even if they are small-scale versions of what Cisco and Dell are trying to do. You just might find that you can be paid to start rock climbing or can gain benefits and perks that go way beyond what's found in the usual job description.

It's quite telling that in a recent poll, 81 percent of those with Internet access across developed nations used it to search for advice about health, medicines, or medical conditions. The poll also found that 68 percent of those who have access have used the Internet to look for information about specific medicines, and nearly four in ten use it to look for other patients' experiences of a condition. Without a doubt new technologies are helping more people around the world to find out more about their health and to make better-informed decisions, but often their online searches lack usefulness because the information retrieved cannot be personalized. Relying on dodgy information can easily lead people to take risks with inappropriate tests and treatments, wasting money and causing unnecessary worry. But with a health-record system like Dell's and its developing infrastructure to tailor health advice and guidance to individual people based on their personal records, the outcome could be revolutionary to our health-care system, instigating the reform that's sorely needed.

Information technology changed the Internet, so now it's time for IT to change medicine, which will in turn change our personal and collective health care. I mean that literally and figuratively. It will change our health-care system, and it will change each of our individual health *care*. After all, you and I are the stakeholders—not the government and not the doctors.

So how do we do this? I believe this will be achieved by our taking charge of personalized medicine, and by creating the quantitative metrics we need to do so. The first baby step rests with each of us: we each need to collect our own data and be the place for data centralization. It's the starting point from which all other roads to health commence. This will allow us to ask the right questions, have the right kind of relationship with our doctor, and participate in the change that will be our health-care reform personalized.

We cannot presume that any health plan proposed or passed for America will improve our health. Yes, it will make more people benefit from health care, but it won't make health care better. We—you and me—need to make health care better by executing the ideas and strategies in this book. After all, the ultimate personal incentive is living as long as we can and as well as we can.

Health Rule

Don't hoard your medical information or keep it secret, as this can ultimately shorten your life and eliminate opportunities to live better and longer. Share it wherever possible, including over the Internet, and be ready to participate in the next revolution that's taking place in medicine. If your employer offers an interactive corporate wellness program, sign up!

14

The Art of Doing Nothing

Honoring Our Body's Natural Healing Powers

Keep to a schedule. Move throughout the day (get out of that chair you are sitting in!). Eat real food to absorb all the nutrition you need. Reduce your daily dose of inflammation. Stay abreast of new technologies that can enhance your health or help you to plan your future health. Share your medical information with the world wherever possible. Those are pretty basic principles. I'll give you one more that will require just a brief explanation: *do nothing*. If there's one thing I've been hinting at throughout this book, it's that the body works in mysterious ways. Often, it can heal on its own when given the chance. In a world where we futilely try to force health on ourselves by taking supplemental vitamins and assuming we need pill A or elixir B, we could potentially do ourselves better once in a while if we did nothing at all.

When I was in training at Johns Hopkins Hospital in Baltimore, a book by Lewis Thomas had a profound effect on me. Thomas was a Renaissance man of sorts, part physician and researcher, part poet and essayist, part educator and administrator, and part policy adviser and mentor. He had a commanding way with words and language—so much so that many described him as the quintessential etymologist. He wrote with such grace, wit, and style that he won a following well beyond the medical profession. In 1974, twenty-nine of his columns that had been published in the *New England Journal of Medicine* monthly since 1971 landed in a book for the lay public called *The Lives of a Cell*, which became a bestseller and was awarded the 1974 National Book Award for Arts and Letters. His stories, originally told as "Notes of a Biology Watcher," present a brief, personal overview of research or a then current subject in the biological sciences. This is scarcely the sort of stuff that would appeal to a wide audience, or so one would think. But the clarity and wisdom with which Thomas wrote found a general audience, partly because his manner was casual, offhand, spontaneous, and richly provocative in subtle ways. He may have authored more than two hundred highly specialized papers in the fields of immunology and pathology, but he is beloved and admired today largely for his informal writings.

I had the privilege to meet Lewis Thomas during my undergraduate years at Princeton in the mid-1980s. I was a junior when they dedicated the new Lewis Thomas laboratories for the Molecular Biology Department, and I was part of the first class to "inhabit" the building. Part of the great benefit of this was to participate in several evening chat sessions with Lewis, which the university arranged for us students. By then Thomas was an elderly, frail man at the tail end of his thriving career, and I was just beginning my studies in molecular biology and medicine. I still remember, though, his simple statement to us all, which I wrote in my calendar then and keep close by to this day: "This is the one chance to learn about other things than medicine. Medicine is the art of observation and interpretation, which are skills that are not learned in a book."

The book that I still hold near and dear to me, as it had an indelible effect on my thinking from those early days of learning my craft, is Thomas's *The Youngest Science: Notes of a Medicine-Watcher*, which was published in 1983. In it, he describes how one of his father's first patients came to him complaining of bloody urine. His father examined the patient and the urine, but couldn't make a diagnosis. To gain time to read up on this and think it through, his father gave the patient a bottle of Blaud's pills, a popular iron treatment for anemia in the 1910s. The patient came back to see his father on the prescribed day and told him that all was perfect—the bloody urine was cured! In all probability, the patient had passed a silent kidney stone or something of that order. But his father's reputation was established. What this story demonstrates is that patients often recover from illnesses without a clear medical explanation. Their bodies heal on their own terms, within their own complex magic, and it's not the doctor that does the saving. Thomas described it beautifully:

> Patients do get better, some of them anyway, from even the worse diseases; there are very few illnesses, like rabies, that kill all comers. Most of them tend to kill some patients and spare others, and if you are one of the lucky ones and have also had at hand a steady, knowledgeable doctor, you become convinced that the doctor saved you. My father's early instructions to me, sitting in the front of his car on his rounds, were that I should be careful not to believe this of myself if I became a doctor.
>
> Nevertheless, despite his skepticism, he carried his prescription pad everywhere and wrote voluminous prescriptions for all his patients. These were fantastic formulations containing five or six vegetable ingredients, each one requiring careful measuring and weighing by the druggist, who pounded the powder, dissolved it in alcohol, and bottled it

with a label giving only the patient's name, the date, and the instructions about dosage. The contents were a deep mystery, and intended to be a mystery. The prescriptions were always written in Latin, to heighten the mystery. The purpose of this kind of therapy was essentially reassurance. . . . They were placebos, and they had been the principal mainstay of medicine, the sole technology, for so long a time—millennia—that they had the incantatory power of religious ritual. My father had little faith in the effectiveness of any of them, but he used them daily in practice. They were expected by his patients; a doctor who did not provide such prescriptions would soon have no practice at all; they did no harm, so far as he could see; if nothing else, they gave the patient something to do while the illness, whatever, was working its way through its appointed course.

The United States Pharmacopoeia, an enormous book, big as the family Bible, stood on a bookshelf in my father's office, along with scores of textbooks and monographs on medicine and surgery. The ingredients that went into the prescriptions, and the recipes for their compounding and administration, were contained in the Pharmacopoeia.

Last year, I purchased a copy of the Pharmacopoeia. Of all places, I found my copy on eBay. What's interesting about this book, aside from the curious and fascinating recipes for treatments, is that its authors convened in 1900 to establish a remarkable set of standards, including nomenclature, units, descriptors, required data elements, and a requirement that every "therapy" included in the compendium be clearly described. The ability of a group of more than a hundred doctors to get together and come to conclusions such as this would be unimaginable today, yet this kind of agreement is sorely needed in health care. The Pharmacopoeia describes how to make thousands of herbal, supplement, and other preparations, though none of the preparations have health claims attached to them, just standardization in their manufacture and preparation. In many respects this book represents the origin of a multibillion-dollar business of vitamins and supplements, although the standardization component seems to have been lost over the years. What's interesting—and troubling—is that vitamins and supplements were in the direct domain of the physician and pharmacists in the early 1900s, and today they have all but vacated the purview of the doctors. Vitamins and supplements aren't even regulated by any governmental or corporate entity to the degree that other, traditional pharmaceutical drugs are.

Like so many other thinkers, doctors, and philosophers that I've referenced in this book, Lewis Thomas's father was insightful beyond his era. He knew that illness carried with it a mysterious serendipity. People can get well for any number of reasons, none of which may be due to any prescribed treatment or "elixir." Indeed, there is something to be said for doing nothing. This isn't meant to discredit known and necessary treatments for certain ailments and diseases, but for purposes of arguing in favor of another perspective, consider, for just a moment, what doing nothing can mean in some other instances. Rather than popping pills and looking for external solutions, you could focus on your body's inherent self-healing mechanisms by regulating it naturally. You could follow the tenets outlined in this book and live in the world of prevention rather than treatment. In doing so, you would honor the body for what it is: a complex, dynamic system that cannot be explained as easily as we'd like it to be. Perhaps you would experience better health in a new and eye-opening way.

Health Rule

Homeostasis is the body's paradise. The body may be complex and hard to fully understand, but it's constantly seeking the simplicity of homeostasis. When we place too many forces on it unnecessarily, such as through drugs, supplements, inconsistent schedules, sleep deprivation, and excessive exercising, eating, or drinking, we break that homeostasis. The good news is we can let our bodies come back to homeostasis naturally just by honoring its preferred rhythms and being mindful of the body's inputs.

Conclusion

Of Mice and Men and the Search for the Master Switch

Do We Have to Die? My Final Notes of Hope

> Healing, Papa would tell me, is not a science, but the intuitive art of wooing nature.
>
> —*W. H. Auden, twentieth-century poet*

Where's the master switch?

It's a good question, one that has swirled around scientific circles for as long as I can remember. Do we need to age? Is there a way to "trick" the body into thinking that it's not getting any older? Can we find the master switch that somehow tells the body to physically begin to turn itself off and prevent that from happening? More to the point, do we need to die?

We may be no better at achieving immortality than our prehistoric ancestors, but we do have a much greater understanding of aging and how to intervene to prolong our lives. We are not only living much longer today, but we're also living much better in those later years than any generation before us. In the last 150 years the average life span has soared from about forty-five to closer to eighty years. Still, we need to, and will, answer myriad questions and conundrums—even if those answers don't lead to immortality. But they will undoubtedly help us to push the boundaries of longevity further—to, as W. H. Auden so terrifically put it, woo nature in our state of perpetual healing.

The idea that all living things have a master switch somewhere deep inside is as fascinating as it is mystical. Consider the following: a mouse will live for about three to five years before getting cancer and dying; a dog will go for about seven to fourteen years before succumbing to that fate; and a human that survives on average into his or her seventh to ninth decade will eventually begin to cancer, barring something else that gets in the way first, such as heart disease or a tragic accident. All three of these species share remarkably similar DNA, but there's a vast difference between living a few years or one decade, and riding into the sunset for nearly a century. Clearly the master switches in the mouse and the dog have different time functions on them than ours do. One day maybe we'll be able to come close to understanding these master switches, or maybe not. Perhaps all we'll be able to do is find ways to control our master switch, which I think is a lot more realistic. It's what I'm attempting to do every single day in my practice and labs.

The end of illness is achievable because of two fundamental beliefs. For one, most diseases are delayable or preventable, and two, a sense of optimism that the "magic pills" to treat many of the ailments of today will be available in the next two decades. I am fortunate to be able to see the progress happening in labs and companies across the world, both on the technology side and drug-development side, and this is where the optimism and hope come from.

That illness is largely preventable cannot be trivialized. This is true even in my line of work. Most cancer deaths are quite avoidable.

If you consider the major killers in men, the top three are prostate, lung, and colon cancer. Together they represent almost 60 percent of deaths from cancer. If you're a man, prostate specific antigen (PSA) tests can identify prostate cancer early through a simple blood sample. If you're at high risk for the disease, you can undergo treatment, whether that means surgery or radiation therapy, that will have a marked effect on your disease's course. The data showing that these interventions actually save lives is not presently available, but I believe it is because these studies take many years to do, and they are currently ongoing. In the case of lung cancer, giving up cigarettes and minimizing your exposure to secondhand smoke can dramatically decrease your risk for this type of cancer, and chest CT screening can decrease your chance of death. Colon cancer can similarly be avoided through colonoscopies that identify polyps prior to their becoming cancerous.

If you're a woman, the top cancer killers are those of the breast, lung, and colon. Again, you can help prevent and treat all of these with current technologies, which have a profound impact on your chances of ever dying from these diseases. Whether you're a man or a woman, preventing heart disease and stroke is also relatively straightforward and actionable. We now know how certain dietary rules and the use of statins where appropriate can come into play. So if you only take a single thing away from this book, let that be the power of preventive medicine. Also bear in mind that this isn't just about you. It's about all of us.

Health-care costs in this country are exorbitant. We spend 17.8 percent of our gross domestic product on health care, which amounts to more than $2 trillion—over four times the amount spent on national defense. This number is predicted to reach 20 percent over the next several years, most of it going to people in their last two years of life. These are the folks who are not living robustly to their last breath; they are sipping expensive air as they loiter in their old age with chronic disease that cannot be managed well or an illness that takes years to fully develop and lead to the inevitable. Health-insurance premiums for an average family continue to rise, costing families who can afford coverage more than $15,000 a year. The US health-care system is broken and is not sustainable. We are presently the highest per capita spender among developed countries. In 2004, we spent approximately 49 percent more than Norway, which spends the third most of developed countries. We are spending two and a half times what the average developed country spends per capita for health care. But our outcomes aren't any better.

Our higher costs have not been linked with better care or safety. Estimates are that 98,000 to 195,000 people per year are presently killed by medical mistakes; 57,000 individuals are estimated to die from inadequate care. Enormous variations in cost can exist within the United States, despite similar quality, and we are ranked thirty-seventh in overall health-system performance by the World Health Organization, yet we are presently number one in spending. We are twenty-second in life expectancy among the thirty developed countries. We have over 50 million uninsured individuals, and over 25 million individuals underinsured, most of whom are working.

The news worsens when we visit the current state of pharmaceuticals. I firmly believe that innovation will save health care—innovation that can empower the individual in the ways I describe in this book, and innovation at places where drug development takes place. The 1980s were a roaring era for drug development thanks to the intrepid lobbying for treatments for HIV/AIDS. But in the following decades, we lost momentum. Back then, fifteen to twenty new chemical entities were developed each year as we wrestled with gaining the upper hand on HIV and other newsworthy diseases; now that number has dwindled to a scant single digit every year. And that's not referring to chemicals targeted at HIV—that's the overall "progress" that we clock annually in all drug development.

Once HIV became a managed condition that wasn't necessarily going to swallow the world's population by storm, we stopped being so vocal and fierce about its research—and all other medical research suffered as a consequence. President Richard Nixon may have declared a "war on cancer" in 1971, but this war is without end, and we seem to have abandoned the front. Since the signing of the National Cancer Act of 1971, we've lost more than 12 million Americans to cancer. Every time a citizen pays $10 in taxes, only one penny goes to cancer research; we allocate less than $5 billion yearly for cancer research while Americans spend $20 billion a year on beauty products, and $5.3 billion on potato chips! We lose roughly 560,000 people a year to cancer, which is 160,000 more than lost their lives in World War II. If health care spending consumes 20 percent of our gross domestic product, why aren't we allocating more money to help ourselves escape this disease that's ravaging our population? But, as I stated once before, this isn't just about cancer. Because cancer is the ultimate nemesis, anything we learn about cancer will benefit all other illnesses. This is especially important at this juncture in human history because alarms have been sounding in many corners of medicine to alert us that some of our oldest nemeses—ones we had thought vanquished—are coming back to haunt us.

Earlier in this book, I may have implied that infectious diseases are relatively "easy" to treat because they involve foreign invaders toward which we can direct lots of effective bullets. But some infections still loom large despite our guns. Barely any doctors still practicing can remember life before antibiotics, when people were routinely hospitalized for common infections, and the threat of deadly *Staphylococcus* shadowed even the simplest surgery. But infectious-disease specialists have been reading up on those days because of a growing fear that rogue bacteria are once again a dire threat. Wealthy countries take for granted the triumph of science over bacteria, but increasingly doctors are battling infections that can only be quelled by the most powerful antibiotics known to medicine—or, at worst, by none of them at all. In the United States alone, antibiotic-resistant infections cause roughly 100,000 deaths a year. Imagine a world in which antibiotics resemble chemotherapy drugs—producing toxic side effects and unpredictable outcomes instead of the guaranteed cures we have come to expect—and you can understand what keeps epidemiologists awake at night. We must respect the complex systems among our fellow organisms, and bacteria are no exception. They will do what live organisms do best: evolve and adapt to new environments.

In addition to society's overuse and abuse of antibiotics, which has led to resistant strains, the rise of these superbugs can partly be blamed on neglect in the crusade for new antibiotics. I've been painting a bright and optimistic picture of medicine's current technologies in rapid development, but we still need more champions of medical innovation if we're going to realize any of these promising breakthroughs soon. Virtually all areas of medicine ache for more brainpower and human capital. Most children today don't grow up wanting to be doctors and researchers; they dream of being the next Internet sensation. Sadly, and in part because of the lack of recent game-changing discoveries, medicine has lost much of its luster. The good news, which I'm putting my trust in, is that the advances already taking place thanks to new technologies will reinvigorate the medical field, making it again a place where participants stand a chance to transform the world.

Claim Your Right to Health

The concept of "rights" is very much at the forefront of our mind-set. We all cherish the right to free speech, the right to privacy, and the right to vote, among others. These are fundamental to the American way of life. But what about the right to health? What about the right to a long, disease-free life?

America has always been rooted in the belief that each person can create his or her own success. We love being independent—the rights of the individual are very much enmeshed in our culture. Independence Day is one of our finest national holidays and a cornerstone of the American psyche. But somehow, that idea of personal independence gets lost once we hit the topic of health. When our health takes a turn or our insurance isn't there when we need it, we like to point a finger elsewhere rather than hold up a mirror. We forget that our founding fathers tried everything in their power to ensure that we would thrive in independence, which I would think entails a great deal of personal integrity, fortitude, and *responsibility*.

I've been drilling the importance of personal responsibility into your head since the beginning of this book, and I want it to be firmly planted in your mind as you move forward now and take the action you need to control your health and life. Every January first, if you want to make just one New Year's resolution that's actually doable, incredibly powerful, and sustainable for the entire year, make it your goal to take full responsibility for your health every single day no matter what life throws at you. If there is a master switch somewhere inside you, only you can ultimately control it.

I once gave a talk at my daughter's school in front of a bunch of sixth-graders. I used an analogy that worked perfectly for this group, who were just beginning to understand what a cell is. In explaining the cell, I asked the kids how they would stop a runaway train. Virtually all of them got the answer right: they'd find the brake. I reminded them that to do this they didn't need to know the nuts-and-bolts workings of a train, or how many pounds of pressure the brakes would apply to make the stop, or even how the brakes worked. Pulling (or pushing or pressing or whatever) on the brake is all that's required. Which is exactly what should happen in taking care of the body. To some degree, science is building the tracks for our trains to run on. But until we can fully understand how our bodies—our individual trains—prefer to operate, we have to do what we can to optimize their functionality. We have to at least be aware of their brakes and accelerators and find ways to manipulate those buttons using the knowledge that we currently have. This will help each of us to gain as much control over that elusive master switch as humanly possible.

My hope is that I've given you plenty of ideas to at least begin to make a tremendous difference in your life. I don't expect you to execute all of the strategies in this book today or to change your lifestyle overnight. More than anything else, getting this far in the book means you've gained an awareness that puts you in a select group of people. That awareness alone will help you make the needed changes to live a more conscious, fulfilling life that will endure the test of time and aging.

I know the value that being healthy brings to people because I see it day in and day out. I also see what sickness can do to people, no matter how much success they have experienced in life or how many, and how deeply, people love them. Without your health, you have nothing. But when you do have good health, pretty much anything is possible. I avoided making big specific claims at the beginning of this book about what following its advice could help you achieve in addition to overall wellness, such as losing weight, improving your appearance, boosting your mind and memory, lifting your spirits, and even enhancing your sex life. I didn't want to identify any single benefit to taking this book's message to heart because the benefits are wide-reaching and of course can differ from person to person. Things tend to fall into place when you're healthy, especially when you approach your health from the systemic perspective that I've been detailing. As Plato once said, "The part can never be well unless the whole is well." Whatever you hope to gain from reading this book, whether you are well or ill, I hope that you at least embrace its call to personal action. The end of illness resides within all of us. It's up to each of us to do what we can to put an end to it. For those who have the courage to join the revolution currently taking place in medicine, I welcome you.

Acknowledgments

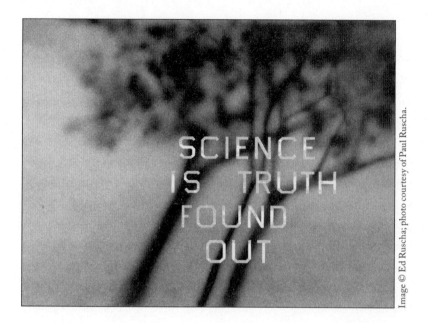

Image © Ed Ruscha; photo courtesy of Paul Ruscha.

At the funeral of Dennis Hopper in June 2010, I asked Ed Ruscha about one of his paintings that had made a tremendous impact on me. The painting states in block letters "SCIENCE IS TRUTH FOUND OUT." I asked Ed why he chose that particular statement, and he responded that he was struck by the saying, which he had first noticed above the entrance to the science lab at Hollywood High School. Scientists, physicians, and researchers all strive to find truth. The path to this truth can be circuitous, many times yielding wrong turns, but the motivation in the health field is to help people live better and longer lives. It is not just a privilege, but also a responsibility to strive for this truth. I have never been on this path alone, and have many to thank.

An entire book could be filled with the names of those who have shaped who I am today, for I owe everyone I've ever worked with and treated through the years a heartfelt thank-you. I especially give a resounding thanks to my patients, who teach me daily about how the body works. If you speak with any of my patients, they will surely tell you they have heard the stories and messages of this book time and time again. Thank you for helping me to hone my message, to continually question and learn about the mysteries of health, and most important, for inviting me to participate in your care; it has been a true honor.

This book reflects the culmination of not just my lifetime work in the health-care industry, but also my ongoing collaboration with a team, and I have many members of the team to thank. First, I have to thank my collaborator, Kristin Loberg. She is a fantastic partner, an insightful thinker, and a good friend. I would like to thank her family, Lawrence and Colin (who was born during the writing of the book), for allowing me to spend the precious time with her over the past two years. To my lawyers, Robert Barnett and David Povich, thank you for doing what you do. You have both been extraordinary in looking after me.

To the excellent team at Free Press whose support and faith made this book possible. Thanks especially to our leader, Dominick Anfuso, and his indefatigable assistant, Maura O'Brien, and to Martha Levin, Carisa Hays, Nancy Inglis, Steve Boldt, Eric Fuentecilla, Larry Hughes, Carla Jones, Suzanne Donahue, Anne Blake, Tracy Lorenzo, Rachel Huffine, and Jennifer Weidman. Thank you for putting up with my constant queries and for hand-holding a new author expertly through the process. To the marketing team of Lynn Goldberg and Megan Beatie at Goldberg McDuffie Communications: you have been tremendous advocates and have championed the message of this book beyond my expectations. Thank you.

In my twenty-one years of training I have been fortunate to work with great mentors and friends. Together you have helped me mature into the physician I have become. Specifically, David Golde, for taking me under your wing; I often wish today you were still here so that I could pick up the phone and once again seek your counsel. To Andy Grove for inspiring me to take greater risks in my thinking and career choices. To my dad for always modeling to me how to be as loving and attentive a doctor as a father. To Steven Spielberg, for your contagious passion and insight. To Larry Ellison, for your certainty and trust in me. To Marc Benioff, for your true friendship. To Al Gore, for pushing me in the right direction (and first introducing me to Danny Hillis). To Max Nikias, Carmen Puliafito, and Eli Broad, for bringing me to USC, a remarkable academic home. To Sumner Redstone, for your unwavering belief in me. To Larry Norton, Danny Hillis, and Murray Gell-Mann, for making me think beyond my own discipline and putting up with my endless questions. To Lance Armstrong and the late Steve Jobs, for your unending inspiration. To Michael Milken and Stuart Holden for your encouragement over the past decade. To John Doerr and Mark Kvamme, for supporting my beliefs and me through the years. To Yossi Vardi and Joe Schoendorf for opening my eyes to health and technology outside the US. To Dan Case, Dennis Hopper, Raul Walters, and Johnny Ramone for teaching me to never give up. To Bill Campbell, for your coaching. And to the team at the USC Westside Cancer Center and Center for Applied Molecular Medicine, particularly Autumn, Justine, Parag, Jonathan, Lisa, Adam, Olga, and Mitchell. Thank you for your loyalty and friendship though the years and thank you for taking this journey with me.

To the many readers of the many drafts of this manuscript. Your encouragement, enthusiasm, and knowledge helped this book take shape. I want to especially thank Marc Benioff, Amy DuRoss, Melissa Floren, Steve Jobs, Avram Miller, Amy Povich, Maury Povich, Dov Seidman, Greg Simon, Bonnie Solow, Elle Stephens, and David N. Weissman.

To my family, you are my true love and passion. Sydney and

Miles, I love you both dearly and can't thank you enough for all your enthusiasm in wanting me to write this book. To my beautiful wife, friend, and partner, Amy, thank you for your influence over me, you have made me a much better person and doctor.

And last, but certainly not least, to you the reader. Thanks for taking the time to think about a whole new way to make this world a better, healthier place.

David B. Agus, M.D.
Beverly Hills, CA

Recommended Reading

The following is a partial list of books and scientific papers that you might find helpful in learning more about some of the ideas and concepts expressed in this book. This is by no means an exhaustive list, but it will get you started in taking a new perspective and in living up to the principles of *The End of Illness*. These materials can also open other doors for further research and inquiry. For access to more studies and an ongoing updated list of references, please visit www.TheEnd ofIllness.com. If you do not see a reference listed here that was mentioned in the book, please refer to the website, where a more comprehensive list is found.

Agus, D.B. et al. Vitamin C crosses the blood-brain barrier in the oxidized form through the glucose transporters. *Journal of Clinical Investigation* 100, no. 11 (1997): 2842–48.

Agus, D.B., J. Vera, and D. Golde. Stromal cell oxidation: A mechanism by which tumors obtain vitamin C. *Cancer Research* 59, no. 18 (1999): 4555–58.

Armstrong, L. *It's Not About the Bike: My Journey Back to Life*. New York: Berkley, 2001.

Atkinson, G., and L. Speirs. Diurnal variation in tennis service. *Perceptual & Motor Skills* 86, no. 3 pt. 2 (June 1998): 1335–38.

Baxter, C., and T. Reilly. Influence of time of day on all-out swimming. *British Journal of Sports Medicine* 17, no. 2 (June 1983): 122–27.

Bishop, D. The effects of travel on team performance in the Australian national netball competition. *Journal of Sports Science and Medicine* 7, no. 1 (March 2004): 118–22.

Bjelakovic, G., D. Nikolova, L.L. Gluud, R.G. Simonetti, and C. Gluud. Mortality in randomized trials of antioxidant supplements for primary and secondary prevention: systematic review and meta-analysis. *Journal of the American Medical Association* 297, no. 8 (February 28, 2007): 842–57.

Recommended Reading

Blair, S.N. Physical inactivity: the biggest public health problem of the 21st century. *British Journal of Sports Medicine* 43, no. 1 (January 2009): 1–2.

Blair, S.N., et al. A tribute to Professor Jeremiah Morris: the man who invented the field of physical activity epidemiology. *Annals of Epidemiology* 20, no. 9 (September 2010): 651–60.

Breus, M. *Good Night: The Sleep Doctor's 4-Week Program to Better Sleep and Better Health.* New York: Dutton, 2006.

Breus, M. *The Sleep Doctor's Diet Plan: Lose Weight through Better Sleep.* Emmaus: Rodale, 2011.

Carney, C.E., J.D. Edinger, B. Meyer, L. Lindman, and T. Istre. Daily activities and sleep quality in college students. *Chronobiology International* 23, no. 3: 623–37.

Center, J.R., D. Bliuc, N.D. Nguyen, T.V. Nguyen, and J.A. Eisman. Osteoporosis medication and reduced mortality risk in elderly women and men. *Journal of Clinical Endocrinology & Metabolism* 96, no. 4 (April 2011): 1006–14. Epub February 2, 2011.

Copinschi, G. Metabolic and endocrine effects of sleep deprivation. *Essential Psychopharmacology* 6, no. 6 (2005): 341–47.

de Lorgeril, M., et al. Cholesterol lowering, cardiovascular diseases, and the rosuvastatin-JUPITER controversy: a critical reappraisal. *Archives of Internal Medicine* 170, no. 12 (June 28, 2010): 1032–36.

Dreyfuss, J.H. Oral bisphosphonate use associated with a decreased risk of breast cancer. *CA—A Cancer Journal for Clinicians* 60, no. 6 (November-December 2010): 343–44. Epub October 19, 2010.

Edwards, B.J., W. Edwards, J. Waterhouse, G. Atkinson, and T. Reilly. Can cycling performance in an early morning, laboratory-based cycle time-trial be improved by morning exercise the day before? *International Journal of Sports Medicine* 26, no. 8 (October 2005): 651–6. Erratum in: *Journal of the American College of Cardiology* 57, no.16 (April 19, 2011): 1717.

FDA website: http://www.fda.gov/food/foodsafety/product-specificinforma tion/seafood/foodbornepathogenscontaminants/methylmercury/ ucm115644.htm.

Forrester, D.P. *Consider: Harnessing the Power of Reflective Thinking in Your Organization.* New York: Palgrave Macmillan, 2011.

Freedman, D.M., A.C. Looker, C.C. Abnet, M.S. Linet, and B.I. Graubard. Serum 25-hydroxyvitamin D and cancer mortality in the NHANES III study (1988–2006). *Cancer Research* 70, no. 21 (November 1, 2010): 8587–97. Epub September 16, 2010.

Garry, A., D.H. Edwards, I.F. Fallis, R.L. Jenkins, and T.M. Griffith. Ascorbic acid and tetrahydrobiopterin potentiate the EDHF phenomenon by generating hydrogen peroxide. *Cardiovascular Research* 84, no. 2 (November 1, 2009): 218–26. Epub July 10, 2009.

Gershon, M. *The Second Brain: The Scientific Basis of Gut Instinct and a Groundbreaking New Understanding of Nervous Disorders of the Stomach and Intestines.* New York: HarperCollins, 1998.

Ginsberg, J., et al. Detecting influenza epidemics using search engine query data. *Nature* 457, no. 7232 (February 2009): 1012–14.

Gnant, M., et al. Endocrine therapy plus zoledronic acid in premenopausal breast cancer. *New England Journal of Medicine* 360, no. 7 (2009): 679–91.

Green, R.C., et al. Disclosure of APOE genotype for risk of Alzheimer's disease. *New England Journal of Medicine* 361, no. 3 (July 16, 2009): 245–54.

Guevara-Aguirre, J., et al. Growth hormone receptor deficiency is associated with a major reduction in pro-aging signaling, cancer, and diabetes in humans. *Science Translational Medicine* 3, no. 70 (February 16, 2011): 70ra13.

Haldane, J.B.S. Daedalus, or Science and the Future. A paper read to the Heretics, Cambridge, UK, February 4, 1923. Transcribed by CR Shalizi, April 10, 1993, Berkeley, CA. Source: http://www.cscs.umich.edu/~crshalizi/daedalus.html.

Hillis, D. TED talk, 2010. Understanding Cancer through Proteomics. Accessed on October 18, 2011. http://www.ted.com/talks/danny_hillis_two_frontiers_of_cancer_treatment.html.

Jablonski, N.G., and G. Chaplin. Colloquium Paper: Human skin pigmentation as an adaptation to UV radiation. *Proceedings of the National Academy of Sciences* 107, Suppl. 2 (May 11, 2010): 8962–68.

Jehue, R., D. Street, and R. Huizenga. Effect of time zone and game time changes on team performance: National Football League. *Medicine & Science in Sports & Exercise* 25, no. 1 (January 1993): 127–31.

Kirsh, V.A., et al. Supplemental and dietary vitamin E, beta-carotene, and vitamin C intakes and prostate cancer risk. *Journal of the National Cancer Institute* 98, no. 4 (February 15, 2006): 245–54.

Klein, E.A., et al. Vitamin E and the risk of prostate cancer: the Selenium and Vitamin E Cancer Prevention Trial (SELECT). *Journal of the American Medical Association* 306, no. 14 (October 12, 2011): 1549–56.

Levitt, S.D., and S.L. Dubner. *Freakonomics: A Rogue Economist Explores the Hidden Side of Everything.* New York: William Morrow, 2006.

Lind, J. *A Treatise on the Scurvy.* Nabu Press, 2011; originally published in 1753.

Manber, R., R.R. Bootzin, C. Acebo, M.A. Carskadon. The effects of regularizing sleep-wake schedules on daytime sleepiness. *Sleep* 19, no. 5 (June 1996): 432–41.

Martí, O., and A. Armario. Influence of regularity of exposure to chronic stress on the pattern of habituation of pituitary-adrenal hormones, prolactin and glucose. *Stress* 1, no. 3 (May 1997): 179–89.

Miller, E.R., 3rd, et al. Meta-analysis: high-dosage vitamin E supplementation may increase all-cause mortality. *Annals of Internal Medicine* 142, no. 1 (January 4, 2005): 37–46. Epub November 10, 2004.

Morris, J.N., and M.D. Crawford. Coronary heart disease and physical activity of work: evidence of a national necropsy survey. *BMJ* 2 (December 20, 1958): 1485–96.

Morris, J.N., J.A. Heady, P.A.B. Raffle, C.G. Roberts, and J.W. Parks. Coronary heart-disease and physical activity of work. *Lancet* 265, no. 6795 (November 21, 1953): 1053–57.

Morris, J.N., J.A. Heady, P.A.B. Raffle, C.G. Roberts, and J.W. Parks. Coronary heart-disease and physical activity of work. *Lancet* 262 (November 28, 1953): 1111–20.

Mukherjee, S. *The Emperor of All Maladies: A Biography of Cancer.* New York: Scribner, 2010.

Neuhouser, M.L., et al. Multivitamin use and risk of cancer and cardiovascular disease in the Women's Health Initiative cohorts. *Archives of Internal Medicine* 169, no. 3 (February 9, 2009): 294–304.

Pollan, M. *In Defense of Food: An Eater's Manifesto.* New York: Penguin, 2009.

Rahman, A.A., et al. Hand pattern indicates prostate cancer risk. *British Journal of Cancer* 104, no. 1 (January 4, 2011): 175–77. Epub November 30, 2010.

Reardon, D.A., et al. A review of VEGF/VEGFR-targeted therapeutics for recurrent glioblastoma. *Journal of the National Comprehensive Cancer Network* 9, no. 4 (April 2011): 414–27.

Rennert, G., et al. Rosuvastatin to prevent vascular events in men and women with elevated C-reactive protein. *New England Journal of Medicine* 359, no. 21 (November 20, 2008): 2195–207. Epub November 9, 2008.

Ridker, P.M.; JUPITER Study Group. Rosuvastatin in the primary prevention of cardiovascular disease among patients with low levels of low-density lipoprotein cholesterol and elevated high-sensitivity C-reactive protein: rationale and design of the JUPITER trial. *Circulation* 108, no. 19 (November 11, 2003): 2292–97.

Rothwell, P.M., et al. Effect of daily aspirin on long-term risk of death due to cancer: analysis of individual patient data from randomised trials. *Lancet* 377, no. 9759 (January 1, 2011): 31–41. Epub December 6, 2010.

Sanders, K.M., et al. Annual high-dose oral vitamin D and falls and fractures in older women: a randomized controlled trial. *Journal of the American Medical Association* 303, no. 18 (2010): 1815–22. doi: 10.1001/jama.2010 .594.

Schrödinger, E. *What Is Life? The Physical Aspect of the Living Cell.* Cambridge, UK: Cambridge Univeristy Press, 1944.

Schürks, M., R.J. Glynn, P.M. Rist, C. Tzourio, and T. Kurth. Effects of vitamin E on stroke subtypes: meta-analysis of randomised controlled trials. *BMJ* 341 (November 4, 2010): c5702. doi: 10.1136/bmj.c5702.

Sedliak, M., T. Finni, S. Cheng, W.J. Kraemer, and K. Häkkinen. Effect of time-of-day-specific strength training on serum hormone concentrations and isometric strength in men. *Chronobiology International* 24, no. 6 (2007): 1159–77.

Snowdon, D. *Aging with Grace: What the Nun Study Teaches Us About Leading Longer, Healthier, and More Meaningful Lives.* New York: Bantam, 2001.

Spiegel, K., et al. Leptin levels are dependent on sleep duration: relationships with sympathovagal balance, carbohydrate regulation, cortisol, and thyrotropin. *Journal of Clinical Endocrinology & Metabolism* 89, no. 11 (November 2004): 5762–71.

Stamatakis, E., M. Hamer, and D.W. Dunstan. Screen-based entertainment time, all-cause mortality, and cardiovascular events: population-based study with ongoing mortality and hospital events follow-up. *Journal of the American College of Cardiology* 57, no. 3 (January 18, 2011): 292–99.

Taheri, S., L. Lin, D. Austin, T. Young, and E. Mignot. Short sleep duration is associated with reduced leptin, elevated ghrelin, and increased body mass index. *PLoS Medicine* 1, no. 3 (December 2004): e62. Epub December 7, 2004.

Thomas, L. *The Lives of a Cell: Notes of a Biology Watcher.* New York: Penguin, 1978.

Virtamo, J., et al. Incidence of cancer and mortality following alpha-tocopherol and beta-carotene supplementation: a postintervention follow-up. *Journal of the American Medical Association* 290, no. 4 (July 23, 2003): 476–85.

Vivekananthan, D.P., M.S. Penn, S.K. Sapp, A. Hsu, and E.J. Topol. Use of antioxidant vitamins for the prevention of cardiovascular disease: meta-analysis of randomised trials. *Lancet* 361, no. 9374 (June 14, 2003): 2017–23.

Wang, T.J., et al. Common genetic determinants of vitamin D insufficiency: a genome-wide association study. *Lancet* 376, no. 9736 (July 17, 2010): 180–88. Epub June 10, 2010.

Zhang, W., et al. Index to ring finger length ratio and the risk of osteoarthritis. *Arthritis & Rheumatism* 58, no. 1 (January 2008): 137–44.

Index

Index

Index

About the Author

Dr. David B. Agus is professor of medicine and engineering at the University of Southern California Keck School of Medicine and the Viterbi School of Engineering and heads USC's Westside Cancer Center and the Center for Applied Molecular Medicine. His research focuses on the application of proteomics and genomics to the study of cancer and the development of new therapeutics for cancer. Dr. Agus received his undergraduate degree from Princeton University and his M.D. from the University of Pennsylvania School of Medicine. Dr. Agus then spent two years at the National Institutes of Health as a Howard Hughes Medical Institute-NIH Research Scholar and did his medical internship and residency training as part of the Osler housestaff at Johns Hopkins Hospital. Dr. Agus completed his oncology fellowship training at Memorial Sloan-Kettering Cancer Center, where later he served as attending physician in the Department of Medical Oncology and as head of the Laboratory of Tumor Biology. He has received various honors and awards including the American Cancer Society Physician Research Award, a Clinical Scholar Award from the Sloan-Kettering Institute, the International Myeloma Foundation Visionary Science Award, and the 2009 *GQ* magazine Rock Star of Science Award. Dr. Agus is an international leader in new technologies and approaches for personalized health care and chairs the Global Agenda Council (GAC) on Genetics for the World Economic Forum. He is the founder of Oncology.com, one of the largest Internet cancer resources and communities, and cofounder of Applied Proteomics and Navigenics, two health-care technology and wellness companies. He lives in California with his wife and two children.

Front cover: An image showing the beautiful richness and complexity of information derived from a drop of human blood. In this new approach to understanding disease, proteins from a blood sample are cut into smaller, more manageable sizes called peptides, which, in their gas state, produce a positive charge that allows them to be manipulated by electrical and magnetic fields. This is what ultimately enables scientists to now "see" and measure certain attributes about all the proteins in the body, which are represented here by the various dots. Technology like this will someday be used to determine the state of your health on a routine basis. At full resolution, this image would have to be printed along the side of a twelve-story building and require using every color the human eye is capable of seeing.